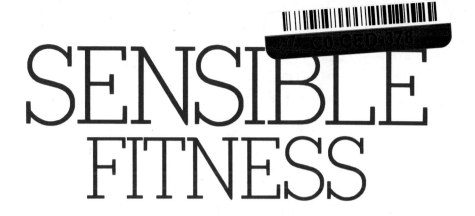

SENSIBLE FITNESS

Second Edition

Jack H. Wilmore, PhD

The University of Texas at Austin

LEISURE PRESS

Champaign, Illinois

Library of Congress Cataloging-in-Publication Data

Wilmore, Jack H., 1938-
    Sensible fitness.

    Rev. ed. of: The Wilmore fitness program. c1981.
    Bibliography: p.
    Includes index.
    1. Physical fitness.   I. Wilmore, Jack H.,
1938-   . Wilmore fitness program. II. Title.
GV481.W564   1986 613.7   85-30927
ISBN 0-88011-270-0

Developmental Editor: Sue Ingels Mauck
Copy Editor: Ann Morris Bruehler
Production Director: Ernie Noa
Typesetter: Yvonne Winsor
Text Layout: Lezli Harris
Cover Design and Layout: Jack Davis
Printed By: United Graphics
Cover Photo: Index Stock International, Inc.
Photo on page 15: used with permission from Gambetta, (Ed.). (1981).
Track and Field Coaching Manual. Champaign, IL: Leisure Press. Page
58: Photo courtesy of Lanie Lass. Page 196: photo used with permission
from Groppel, J.L. (1984). *Tennis for Advanced Players.* Champaign,
IL: Human Kinetics Publishers.

ISBN: 0-88011-270-0

Printed in the United States of America

10 9 8 7 6 5 4 3 2 1

Leisure Press
A division of Human Kinetics Publishers, Inc.
Box 5076, Champaign, IL 61820

To my wife, Dottie

Contents

Acknowledgments

Writing a book involves the efforts of many individuals, most of whom receive little or no recognition. This book would not have been a reality if it weren't for the efforts of the following people. A special thanks to my wife, Dottie, and my daughters, Wendy, Kristi, and Melissa, for their encouragement, and for making sacrifices to allow me time to complete this book; to Mom and Dad for their love and guidance over the years; to my spiritual counselors, Pastors Ron Ritchie, John Dungey, Roger Barrier, and Leonard Karlberg, for their leadership in helping me establish my priorities as a Christian, and in encouraging my spiritual growth; to all of my professional colleagues who have worked so diligently to establish new frontiers in exercise physiology and sports medicine; and to all of my students, past, present, and future, for providing me with the stimulus to continue to learn and to do my best, and who are a continual source of joy and pleasure.

Special recognition goes to Fred Anderson for the outstanding job he did in providing all of the original illustrations for this book; to Christine Coronado for her conscientious efforts in typing the final manuscript; to Phil Stanforth and Tracy Sullivan for serving as models for many of the photographs used in this book; and to all of the people at Leisure Press and Human Kinetics Publishers, who have provided so much help in the final production of this book.

Preface

Research in the sport and exercise sciences has now clearly established the need for a physically active life-style to achieve optimal health and to prevent the early onset of diseases associated with a sedentary existence. In response to this growing body of evidence, Americans have become more aware of their need to be more active. From early childhood to the senior adult, organized programs have been designed and developed to meet the activity needs of the general population. Still, there is considerable misunderstanding as to the specific role exercise plays in promoting health and preventing disease. Further, few understand the principles behind the prescription of exercise for its health-related benefits. It was for these reasons that this book had its initial genesis. First published by Simon and Schuster in 1981, under the title *The Wilmore Fitness Program*, this book has been revised and published by Leisure Press in expectation of reaching an audience that is truly concerned about optimizing their health and productivity.

Jack H. Wilmore
Austin, Texas
October 14, 1985

P A R T

Good Health Through Physical Activity and Sport

The beginning of the twentieth century marked a significant period of transition in the history of the United States. Automobiles, airplanes, radios, movies, and the widespread use of the telephone were the more visible symbols of a society which was becoming highly mechanized. As late as the year 1900, 60% of the American population lived on farms or in towns of less than 4,000 inhabitants, and were dependent directly or indirectly on agriculture for their livelihood. With increased mechanization in an age of modern technology, and the general migration of people into the cities or urban areas where hard physical labor was replaced by occupations of a highly sedentary nature, a new life-style emerged which included little, if any, physical activity.

Have we successfully adapted to this change in life-style? The first chapter of this book attempts to answer this question, focusing on those diseases which have been associated with physical inactivity. The second chapter discusses the implications of a more active life-style relative to health and longevity. In short, Part I of this book describes the health problems associated with our modern life-style, and investigates how increased physical activity through recreational exercises and sport can promote improved health and a sense of well-being.

Diseases and Disability Associated With Physical Inactivity

Since the turn of this century, we have witnessed the transformation of a basically hard-working, physically active, rural-based society into a population of anxious and troubled city dwellers and suburbanites who start to sweat and breathe hard at the mere thought of exercise and vigorous physical activity. Modern technology has made it possible for us to live comfortably with little expenditure of energy. Hand or push lawnmowers were replaced by power lawnmowers, which, in turn, have been replaced by artificial grass. Elevators and escalators have replaced stairs, making it almost impossible to locate an open stairwell in a modern office building, hotel, or department store. Driving has replaced walking, to the point where anxiety and frustration result from being unable to locate a parking space directly in front of the point of destination—even when there are an abundance of parking spaces within a hundred yards or less walking distance. It is a major family tragedy when the remote control for the television set is suddenly in need of repair. While our bodies are crying out for increased opportunities to be physically active, we are continuously looking for ways to make life even easier, conserving effort and human energy. What do we do with all of this effort and energy that we have saved? Or, possibly, we should ask the question: What does a sedentary life-style do to us as individuals? Do we profit, or do we suffer?

The human body is the most complex entity known to man. Scientists have been attempting to unravel the mysteries of the human body for centuries. While great advances have occurred in gaining an understanding of its basic structure and function, we have only started to scratch the surface. If you have ever taken the time to study the human body and how it works, it is impossible not to be impressed with the delicate and intricate manner in which it functions. The various body systems interact in perfect harmony. One slight disruption to any one part generally affects the body as a whole. Hit the end of your finger with a hammer and notice how the pain shoots up your arm and down the back of your legs to your feet! Or, recall the influence on the total body of a simple cold or headache. We are now beginning to realize that physical inactivity is also a stressor to the body, resulting in major deterioration of normal body function. Such common and serious medical problems as coronary heart disease, hypertension, obesity, anxiety and depression, and lower back problems have been either directly or indirectly associated with a lack of physical activity.

In 1961, Drs. Hans Kraus and Wilhelm Raab published a book titled *Hypokinetic Disease*. Several years earlier, Dr. Kraus had coined the Greek composite term "hypokinetic"; "hypo" referring to "less than normal," and "kinetic" referring to "active or dynamic." Thus, *hypokinetic diseases* are those diseases which are associated with less than normal activity, or what has been termed physical inactivity.

Coronary Artery Disease

Of the nearly 2,000,000 deaths which occur each year, 49% of these deaths are the direct result of cardiovascular disease (refer to Figure 1). The major diseases of the cardiovascular system include high blood pressure and stroke, heart attack, congestive heart failure, rheumatic heart disease, and congenital heart defects. Heart attacks alone accounted for 554,900 deaths in 1982 in the United States, which represented 56% of those deaths resulting from cardiovascular disease, or nearly a third of all deaths during that year! In other words, for every three deaths, one was the result of a heart attack.

Heart attacks are the result of *coronary artery disease*, or *atherosclerosis* of the *coronary arteries*. The coronary arteries are those arteries which supply the heart muscle with blood and nutrients, and remove waste products. Atherosclerosis is a slow progressive disease, where the inner lining of the arteries becomes thickened and roughened by deposits of smooth muscle, fat, *fibrin*, cellular debris, and calcium. Figure 2 illustrates the progressive nature of this disease. As the inner lining of the coronary artery becomes more thickened, the area through which the blood can flow is narrowed, making it difficult to meet the demands of the heart when it is under

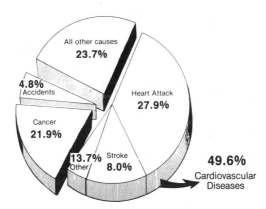

Figure 1   Leading causes of death in the United States in 1982

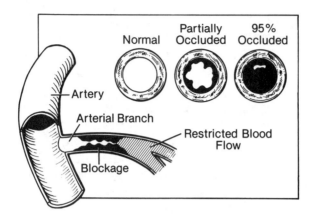

Figure 2   The progressive narrowing of a coronary artery, from a cross-sectional view

stress, such as during exercise. Also, if a clot forms in this area, or if a clot forms in another region and breaks lose and lodges in this narrowed channel, the artery becomes blocked, depriving the heart muscle that it supplies of the necessary nutrients and oxygen. The blockage of a coronary artery precipitates a heart attack, and that portion of the heart muscle that was supplied by that artery beyond the blockage dies (see Figure 3). The greater the area supplied by that artery, the larger the area of heart muscle that dies, and the more severe the resulting heart attack. The left coronary artery, which supplies the left side of the heart, and most importantly the *left ventricle*, is particularly vulnerable. The left ventricle pumps blood through the arterial system, throughout the entire body. Extensive damage to the muscular wall of the left ventricle is quite serious, and frequently results in death.

The narrowing of the coronary arteries is a long and slow process that appears to have its origins early in life. Kannel and Dawber (1972) stated that while atherosclerosis is a disease of the aged, its origins begin in childhood. They cite evidence to indicate that the pathological changes which lead to atherosclerosis begin in infancy and progress during childhood. A study of U.S. Korean War combat casualties, with an average age of 22.1 years, revealed that 77% of these young men had at least moderately advanced coronary atherosclerosis. A more recent study demonstrated evidence of

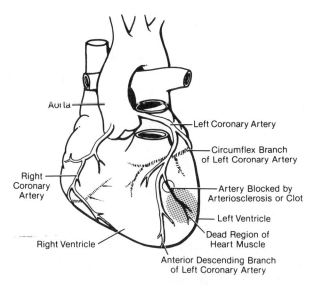

Figure 3 Diagram of the heart and its blood supply through the coronary arteries. Notice the small branch off of the anterior descending branch of the left coronary artery. It has become occluded, resulting in a heart attack, and death of the tissue supplied by that branch.

atherosclerosis in 45% of a group of U.S. Vietnam War combat casualties, with 5% exhibiting severe coronary atherosclerosis. Korean and Vietnamese casualties were found to be relatively free of this disease.

The natural history of atherosclerosis can be divided into three stages: (1) an incubation period which starts early in life and continues throughout adolescence; (2) a latent period that is without symptoms, but in which definite pathological changes can be demonstrated at an early age; and (3) a clinical period during which signs and symptoms first appear.

The incubation period is characterized by fatty streaks in the arterial wall. This is the earliest alteration that can be seen. By the age of 3 years, fatty streaks are present in the *aorta*, the large artery through which the blood leaves the left ventricle of the heart (see Figure 3), of almost all childen regardless of their geographical location or diet. During the latent period, beginning in the second decade, the fatty streaks increase in number, size, and distribution, and first become evident in the coronary arteries. The fatty streak is considered to be reversible with life-style changes including diet and exercise among others. If there is no intervention in the progression of the fatty streak, the most commonly accepted hypothesis suggests that the fatty streak progresses to a *fibrous plaque* during the third decade of life. This stage of development is considered irreversible. The disease reaches the clinical period when the fibrous plaque has progressed to the point where there is significant narrowing of the coronary artery, sufficient to prevent the heart from receiving the blood it needs during periods of stress.

When narrowed coronary arteries prevent enough blood from flowing to the heart, *myocardial ischemia*, or a local and temporary deficiency of blood, occurs. Most individuals who have episodes of myocardial ischemia, usually associated with exertion, have extreme chest discomfort or pain called *angina pectoris*. Often, the pain radiates down the left shoulder and arm, and is usually moderate to extreme in intensity. There is a large percentage of the population, however, which has the same degree of myocardial ischemia, but no associated pain. Approximately 5% to 10% of the "normal" population fall into this category, which is commonly referred to as *"silent heart disease."*

There is still considerable debate as to the cause of coronary artery disease. Many research investigations have been conducted using both animal and human models, yet the disease process is not totally understood. There have been many approaches taken in the study of coronary artery disease, but one of the more interesting and productive approaches, with possible immediate implications, has been the epidemiologic approach. *Epidemiology* is the study of the relationships of factors that determine the frequencies and distributions of a particular infectious disease, process, or physiological state. With respect to coronary artery disease, entire communities or populations have been studied for long periods of time, up to several decades in length. Annual or biannual medical examinations, in addition to comprehensive family and personal medical histories, usually are included in this type of study.

As an example of this approach, in 1949, the National Heart Institute, now the National Heart, Lung, and Blood Institute, began a prospective epidemiological investigation of coronary artery disease in Framingham, Massachusetts, which has become known as the "Framingham Study." Although federal funding of the long-term study was terminated in the early 1970s, the community has continued to support the costs associated with conducting the project, although at a reduced level, to allow continuation of the project. Further government support has been recently obtained for studying the offspring of the original Framingham participants. Over a period of years, many individuals in the community being studied die from a variety of causes, but a substantial number from coronary artery disease. By reviewing the medical histories of those who die from coronary artery disease, it is possible to see what medical abnormalities or problems these individuals have in common. From the Framingham Study, and from similar studies conducted in other communities, a consistent pattern has evolved. A number of factors have been identified, that when present, place the individual at an increased risk for coronary artery disease. These factors include the following:

Factors That Cannot Be Altered
- heredity
- gender
- race
- age

Factors That Can Be Altered

Primary
- cigarette smoking and possibly other tobacco use
- hypertension or high blood pressure
- elevated serum cholesterol, triglycerides, or low density lipoproteins

Secondary
- diet
- obesity
- physical inactivity
- diabetes
- emotional stress and anxiety
- electrocardiogram abnormalities

Of those factors which can be altered, three are considered to be of significantly greater importance, and are referred to as primary risk factors. Cigarette smoking, *hypertension* or high blood pressure, and elevated blood fats are considered by most researchers and clinicians to be the most critical or important risk factors. Figure 4 illustrates the influence of the presence of one or more of the primary risk factors on the increasing risk for heart attack or stroke. It is important to note that someone who has all three primary risk factors is at 5.0 times greater risk for heart attack, and 10.6 times greater risk for stroke than the individual who has none of these three risk factors. It is tempting to postulate that the individual who stops smoking and reduces *cholesterol* and blood pressure to

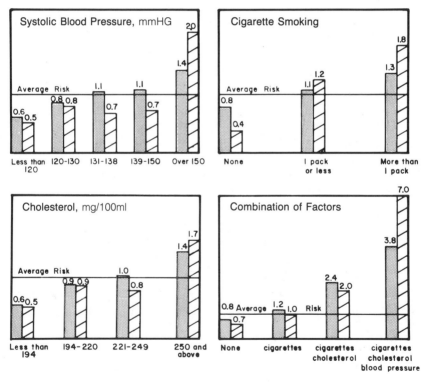

Figure 4 Increased risk of heart attack (open columns) and stroke (hatched columns) with one or more of the primary risk factors. (Data is from the Framingham, Massachusetts, Heart Study.)

normal levels will decrease his or her risk for heart attack and stroke to the level of the individual with no risk factors, but evidence is incomplete at this time. The American Heart Association (1986) has stated that it believes that risk factor modification will reduce the risk for heart attack and stroke to the level of the individual with no risk factors, and that the greatest improvement will result from the simultaneous reduction of all possible factors.

Since research has already demonstrated marked coronary artery disease in young men, it is obvious that a 40- or 50-year-old man who smokes two packs of cigarettes a day, has high blood pressure, and has elevated levels of cholesterol will already have significant narrowing of the coronary arteries. However, it is hoped that altering risk factors by changing one's life-style will alter the course of the disease, or its rate of progression. Research and clinical trials are presently under way in various communities throughout the United States attempting to determine whether risk factor modification does reduce the risk for the disease. The Multiple Risk Factor Intervention Trial (MRFIT) study (1982) investigated the efficacy of altering the three primary risk factors. They randomly assigned 12,866 high-risk men, 35 to 57 years of age, to either an intervention, or risk factor modification group, or to a group that received standard medical care. While both groups decreased risk factor levels over a period of 7 years, the intervention group demonstrated the largest decrease. Interestingly, there were no differences in coronary artery disease deaths over this 7-year period between the two groups. This latter finding was unexpected, and is possibly explained by the fact that both groups decreased their risk factor levels, and the overall mortality for both groups was considerably lower than would have been expected.

It is encouraging to note that there has been a steady decrease in the mortality rate (deaths/100,000 population) for coronary artery disease since the early to mid-1960s. From an epidemic rise in death rate up to 1963, the trend reversed itself, and there has been a decline in coronary artery disease deaths of 3% between 1963 and 1982. Figure 5 illustrates this remarkable trend. While these results are encouraging, it is still unknown if the observed decline in mortality is the result of decreasing numbers of new heart attacks, or to increasing survivorship after developing the disease. There is substantial data available to support the concept that at least part of this decline can be directly linked to the beneficial changes that have taken place in cardiovascular health habits, risk factor modifications, and better medical management of the disease. This downward trend coincides with declines nationally in the percentages of people who smoke, in percentages of people with high cholesterol levels, and in the per capita consumption of eggs, butter, milk, and animal fats. Likewise, there has been a concomitant increase in the recognition and treatment of high blood pressure and in the promotion of a more active life-style.

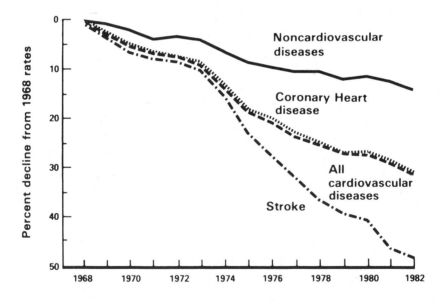

Figure 5   Relative decrease in death rates for cardiovascular and noncardiovascular diseases between the years 1962 and 1982. (From the National Center for Health Statistics.)[1]

[1]Cause of death trends have been adjusted for discontinuities due to revision of International Classification of Diseases.

The American Heart Association (1984) has also made the statement that developing a pattern in early childhood which tends to prevent controllable risk factors from developing is the best way to prevent or delay the onset of heart attack and stroke in later years. It would seem prudent to recommend *avoidance of tobacco, control of blood pressure, control of body weight to a desirable level, eating a well-balanced diet with foods low in saturated fat and cholesterol, regular daily exercise, and a regular medical examination starting at a very early age.* While there is not sufficient "hard" or irrefutable evidence to prove beyond doubt that this course of action will absolutely prevent coronary artery disease, there is a wealth of indirect evidence that would indicate this to be the sound approach to leading a healthy life.

Hypertension

Hypertension is the medical term used to signify a persistently high or elevated blood pressure, above levels considered normal or desirable on the basis of the age of the individual. Blood pressure simply reflects the pressure exerted by the blood on the vessels through which it flows, similar to the way water pressure reflects the pressure of water on the pipes through which it flows. Water pressure is typically constant; you open the faucet and water runs out at a rate dictated by the existing water pressure. Blood pressure does not remain constant, but changes with each beat of the heart. As the heart contracts, it pumps blood out of the heart and into the arteries, thus increasing the pressure within the arteries. This peak pressure, which follows each contraction of the heart, is referred to as the *systolic blood pressure*. As the heart relaxes, preparing for the next contraction, the blood pressure within the artery drops to its lowest level, which is referred to as the *diastolic blood pressure*.

High blood pressure is recognized as a silent, mysterious disease, which kills many thousands of Americans each year. It has no specific warning symptoms, thus millions of Americans have the disease, but have no indication that it is present.

The cause of hypertension is unknown in approximately 90% of those individuals found to be hypertensive, and there is no cure for this disease. Recent research has demonstrated, however, that altered diet, weight reduction, and increased exercise can reduce abnormally elevated blood pressure to normal or near-normal levels. A study by Reisin et al. (1978) found that weight reduction alone had a substantial influence on the reduction of blood pressure in hypertensive patients. Of 57 patients, all but two showed meaningful reductions in blood pressure, and 61% returned to normal blood pressure values. Medication has also been found to be effective in treating hypertension, but, again, hypertension can only be controlled, not cured, so medication would have to be continued indefinitely.

Recent estimates suggest that 13% of the white male, 25% of the black male, 17% of the white female, and 28% of the black female adult population, age 20 years and above, have hypertensive disease. In the year 1982, it was estimated that nearly 38 million Americans had hypertension, but as many as 30% of these, or more, were unaware that they had the disease. What is considered to be abnormally high blood pressure? Most clinicians would agree that a systolic blood pressure in excess of 140 millimeters of mercury, and/or a diastolic pressure in excess of 90 millimeters of mercury would be levels of concern in adults. Levels of concern would be substantially less in children. Periodic blood pressure checks are a very inexpensive form of preventive medicine. It takes only a few minutes of time, and could save a life.

Obesity

It has been stated that obesity is this country's "gross national product." It is true that obesity has become a problem of epidemic proportions in the United States. What a paradox—that while people in many parts of this world are starving to death, we are literally eating ourselves to death! Unfortunately, it is difficult to determine just how many Americans are obese, since *obesity* is defined as being overfat. *Overweight* is defined as exceeding the maximum weight listed by sex, height, and frame size in a table of standard values. Unfortunately, the standard tables represent only average or normative data for the population as a whole, and don't take into consideration the composition of the body. There are many individuals who are overweight on the basis of the standard height-weight tables, yet have a normal or lower than normal amount of body fat. Thus, they are overweight, but not obese (overfat). Many athletes tend to fall into this category as a result of their heavy bones and large muscle mass. Others fall within the prescribed range of weights for their heights and frame size, yet have more than a normal amount of body fat. They would be obese, yet of "normal" weight. Thus, we should concern ourselves with evaluating the degree of obesity of each individual, and not be overly concerned with whether that individual is overweight, underweight, or of normal weight. As an example, in a study we conducted of 180 professional football players, these athletes had an average height of 6 feet, 2 inches, and an average weight of 220 pounds. According to the standard height-weight tables, these athletes should have had an average weight of not more than 194 pounds. Therefore, they were 26 pounds overweight! When we assessed their body composition by techniques to be described later, we found them to have an average of only 13.5% body fat, which is considerably below the average for their age. They were overweight, yet underfat.

How are overweight and obesity assessed? As was mentioned above, overweight simply implies that the individual exceeds a range of weights specified by sex, height, and frame size. The Metropolitan Life Insurance Company of New York developed tables of desirable weights for men and women in the year 1960. Their data was taken from the 1959 Build and Blood Pressure study of the Society of Actuaries. In 1983, the Metropolitan Life Insurance Company released an updated version of these tables, basing the new tables on the 1979 Build and Blood Pressure Study. For the same height and frame size, the new tables allow more weight: 13 and 10 pounds for short men and women, respectively; 7 and 8 pounds for men and women of medium height, respectively; and 2 and 3 pounds for tall men and women, respectively. These new, 1983 tables have received considerable criticism from the scientific medical community. The American Heart Association has recommended the continued use of the 1960 tables. These tables are reproduced in Table 1, and are intended to be used only for those individuals 25 years of age or older. Desirable weight tables are based on the concept that once growth in height stops, there is no biological need for further gains in weight, excluding periods of pregnancy. The weights in these tables were obtained with the individuals wearing shoes and indoor clothing. To translate these figures to nude weights without shoes, you should add one inch for heels in men and two inches for heels in women, and subtract five to seven pounds for clothing. However, the allowance for shoes is almost equally balanced by the allowance for indoor clothing, so the tables can be used directly, that is, with your actual height in bare feet and your nude weight, with little or no loss in accuracy.

When using tables such as these to determine desirable weights, it is necessary to know your frame size. Unfortunately, when these tables were originally developed, there was no indication given as to how to estimate frame size. Subsequent attempts have met with little success. It can only be assumed that those with thick chests, broad shoulders, broad hips, and large or thick wrists are to be considered as large-framed, and those with thin chests, narrow shoulders, narrow hips, and small or thin wrists are considered small-framed, with those in between to be considered as medium-framed. Unfortunately, too many individuals use frame size to justify their present weight. It is interesting to note that while bone size remains stable once one reaches maturity, the frame size tends to increase from small to medium, and then medium to large, in direct proportion to one's increase in body weight over the years.

How accurate are these tables for determining one's ideal or desirable weight? If you happen to fall directly at the midpoint of the population for your height, the tables will be adequate. Unfortunately, few people represent the average for the population, thus the tables can be in error for a substantial percentage of the population. The standard tables only allow you to compare your weight against the normal values for that segment of the male or female adult population that has the

Table 1 Desirable Weights for Men and Women, 25 Years of Age and Over (From the Metropolitan Life Insurance Company of New York, 1960)

Height Feet Inches		Small Frame	Medium Frame	Large Frame
MEN				
5	2	112-120	118-129	126-141
5	3	115-123	121-133	129-144
5	4	118-126	124-136	132-148
5	5	121-129	127-139	135-152
5	6	124-133	130-143	138-156
5	7	128-137	134-147	142-161
5	8	132-141	138-152	147-166
5	9	136-145	142-156	151-170
5	10	140-150	146-160	155-174
5	11	144-154	150-165	159-179
6	0	148-158	154-170	164-184
6	1	152-162	158-175	168-189
6	2	156-167	162-180	173-194
6	3	160-171	167-185	178-199
6	4	164-175	172-190	182-204

Height Feet Inches		Small Frame	Medium Frame	Large Frame
WOMEN				
4	10	92- 98	96-107	104-119
4	11	94-101	98-110	106-122
5	0	96-104	101-113	109-125
5	1	99-107	104-116	112-128
5	2	102-110	107-119	115-131
5	3	105-113	110-122	118-134
5	4	108-116	113-126	121-138
5	5	111-119	116-130	125-142
5	6	114-123	120-135	129-146
5	7	118-127	124-139	133-150
5	8	122-131	128-143	137-154
5	9	126-135	132-147	141-158
5	10	130-140	136-151	145-163
5	11	134-144	140-155	149-168
6	0	138-148	144-159	153-173

same height and frame size. Considering the inaccuracies of these tables on the basis of their inability to differentiate the composition of the body, that is, bone, muscle, and fat, and the fact that for any one category of height and frame size the weights will range from 7 to 24 pounds, one must conclude that the standard tables for determining desirable weight are of little value in helping us each determine our best or ideal body weight.

What are the alternatives, if any? The actual amount of fat weight and *lean body weight* (muscle, bone, organs, skin, etc.) can be determined in the laboratory through various scientific techniques. The most widely used technique, and possibly the most accurate technique, is the *hydrostatic weighing* technique, where the individual is weighed while totally submerged underwater. The weight is taken at that point when the individual has exhaled all of the air out of the lungs (Figure 6). This weight is then corrected for the buoyancy effect of additional air trapped in the lungs and pockets of gas in the stomach and intestines.

How does the above relate to body composition? The density of pure fat is substantially less than the density of water, thus fat will float on water. The density of the lean tissue is substantially above that of water. In simple terms, an obese individual with a large amount of body fat will have a low body density, and will float with ease when placed into a swimming pool. The lean individual with small amounts of body fat will have a high body density, and will find it nearly impossible to float when placed into that same swimming pool. As a second illustration, taking two men of exactly the same height and weight, but one is very fat and the other is very lean, the fat individual will weigh much less than the lean individual when weighed underwater, even though their actual weights are identical.

From body density, equations have been established over the years which allow the estimation of *relative body fat*, or that percentage of the total body weight which is fat. As an example, an individual who weighed 200 pounds and was determined to be 20% body fat would have 40 pounds of fat (200 pounds × 20%) and 160 pounds of lean tissue (200 pounds − 40 pounds of fat). Is 20% too high, too low, or just right?

Figure 6 The hydrostatic weighing technique, to determine body composition

The answer to this question depends only on your sex. Men should be between 12% and 17% body fat, while women should be between 19% and 24% body fat. Any value in excess of 25% body fat for men and 30% body fat for women would be considered obese, and any value in between 20% and 25% for men and 25% to 30% for women would be considered borderline obesity. To determine the ideal or desirable body weight for an individual, you simply divide the individual's lean body weight by that fraction of his or her weight that you want to be lean.

Table 2 should provide a summary of everything discussed above. Mr. Jones and Mr. Smith come to the University of Texas to have their ideal body weight determined. By weighing them underwater, the following values are ob-

Table 2 Determining Ideal Body Weight in Two Men of Identical Weight

Values Assessed	Mr. Jones		Mr. Smith	
Age, years	45		42	
Height	70.0 in	177.8 cm	70.0 in	177.8 cm
Weight	195.0 lb	88.4 kg	195.0 lb	88.4 kg
Underwater weight		5.5 kg		2.5 kg
Volume (weight – underwater weight)		82.9 kg		85.9 kg
Density (mass or weight/volume)		1.066 gm/ml		1.029 gm/ml
Relative Fat		14.2%		31.0%
Fat weight (relative fat × 's weight)	27.7 lb	12.6 kg	60.4 lb	27.4 kg
Lean body weight (total weight – fat weight)	167.3 lb	75.8 kg	134.6 lb	61.0 kg
Ideal weight (lean body weight/0.85[1])	197.0 lb	89.2 kg	158.3 lb	71.8 kg
Weight loss (total weight – ideal weight)	none		37.0 lb	16.6 kg

[1]0.85 is the fractional equivalent of 85%, which represents the stated desired fraction of the total body weight constituted by the lean body weight.

tained, assuming that 15% body fat or 85% lean body weight is the desired body composition.

From this example, it is obvious that Mr. Jones is heavily muscled and probably large boned, while Mr. Smith is obese. While they weigh the same at the present time, Mr. Jones is already below his projected weight for 15% body fat, while Mr. Smith will have to lose 37 pounds to get to his desired weight of 158 pounds. According to Table 1, both men are equally overweight by a minimum of 21 pounds if they were considered to be of large frame. The relative body fat values for male and female athletes in various sports are presented in Table 3, to illustrate the wide range of values in a group of individuals who are considered to be in optimal health.

Table 3   Percentage Body Fat in Male and Female Athletes

Athletic Group or Sport	Males	Females
Baseball	10-15	—
Basketball	7-12	18-27
Canoeing	10-14	—
Football	8-18	—
Gymnastics	3- 6	8-18
Ice hockey	12-16	—
Jockeys	6-16	—
Skiing		
Alpine	10-17	—
Cross-country	7-13	18-24
Nordic	8-14	—
Ski-jumping	12-16	—
Soccer	7-12	—
Speed-skating	8-14	—
Swimming	4-10	12-20
Track and Field		
Runners	4-12	8-18
Jumpers/Hurdlers	—	12-22
Discus	12-18	22-28
Shot Put	14-20	23-30
Tennis	12-16	—
Volleyball	—	20-23
Weight lifting	6-16	—
Wrestling	6-12	—

Obviously, it would be impossible to weigh the entire population of the United States underwater to determine actual body fat levels, so what are the alternatives? The most accurate of the alternatives uses a skinfold caliper to measure the thickness of two layers of skin and the layer of fat which is interposed between the layers of skin. Measurements are taken at six different sites and the resulting values are summed and are used to estimate relative body fat through a series of equations. Tables 4, 5, and 6 provide estimates of relative body fat from the sum of six skinfolds. Figures 7 through 12 illustrate the technique for obtaining accurate skinfold measurements at the specific sites.

Another technique which can be used by anyone who doesn't have access to a skinfold caliper or to an underwater weighing facility employs only a tape measure. For men, the circumference of the waist, exactly at the level of the umbilicus, or belly button, is measured with the tape held firmly in the horizontal position; do not allow the tape to slope upward or downward. The resulting measurement is used to estimate

Figure 7 Skinfold measurement at the triceps site

Figure 8 Skinfold measurement at the scapula site

Figure 9 Skinfold measurement at the chest site.

Figure 10 Skinfold measurement at the suprailiac site.

Figure 11 Skinfold measurement at the abdominal site.

Figure 12 Skinfold measurement at the thigh site.

Table 4 Relative Body Fat From the Sum of Six Skinfolds[1] in Adult Women (in mm)

Sum of 6 Skinfolds	Age to Last Year								
	18 to 22	23 to 27	28 to 32	33 to 37	38 to 42	43 to 47	48 to 52	53 to 57	58 and older
38- 42	11.0	11.2	11.3	11.5	11.6	11.8	11.9	12.1	12.2
43- 47	12.3	12.4	12.6	12.7	12.9	13.0	13.2	13.3	13.5
48- 52	13.5	13.7	13.8	14.0	14.1	14.3	14.4	14.6	14.7
53- 57	14.7	14.9	15.0	15.2	15.3	15.5	15.6	15.8	15.9
58- 62	15.9	16.1	16.2	16.4	16.5	16.7	16.8	17.0	17.1
63- 67	17.1	17.2	17.4	17.5	17.7	17.8	18.0	18.1	18.3
68- 72	18.2	18.3	18.5	18.6	18.8	19.0	19.1	19.3	19.4
73- 77	19.3	19.4	19.6	19.7	19.9	20.1	20.2	20.4	20.5
78- 82	20.4	20.5	20.7	20.8	21.0	21.1	21.2	21.4	21.6
83- 87	21.4	21.6	21.7	21.9	22.0	22.2	22.3	22.5	22.6
88- 92	22.4	22.6	22.7	22.9	23.0	23.2	23.4	23.5	23.7
93- 97	23.4	23.6	23.7	23.9	24.0	24.2	24.3	24.5	24.7
98-102	24.4	24.6	24.7	24.9	25.0	25.2	25.3	25.5	25.6
103-107	25.4	25.5	25.7	25.8	26.0	26.1	26.3	26.4	26.6
108-112	26.3	26.4	26.6	26.7	26.8	27.0	27.2	27.3	27.5

(Cont.)

Table 4 (Cont.)

113-117	27.2	27.3	27.5	27.6	27.8	27.9	28.1	28.2	28.4
118-122	28.0	28.2	28.3	28.5	28.6	28.8	28.9	29.1	29.2
123-127	28.9	29.0	29.2	29.3	29.5	29.6	29.8	29.9	30.1
128-132	29.7	29.8	30.0	30.1	30.3	30.4	30.6	30.7	30.8
133-137	30.5	30.6	30.8	30.9	31.1	31.2	31.4	31.5	31.7
138-142	31.2	31.4	31.5	31.7	31.8	32.0	32.1	32.3	32.4
143-147	31.9	32.1	32.2	32.4	32.6	32.7	32.8	33.0	33.2
148-152	32.6	32.8	33.0	33.1	33.3	33.4	33.6	33.7	33.9
153-157	33.3	33.5	33.6	33.8	33.9	34.1	34.2	34.4	34.5
158-162	34.0	34.1	34.3	34.4	34.6	34.7	34.8	35.0	35.2
163-167	34.6	34.8	34.9	35.1	35.2	35.4	35.5	35.7	35.8
168-172	35.2	35.4	35.5	35.7	35.8	36.0	36.1	36.3	36.4
173-177	35.8	35.9	36.1	36.2	36.4	36.5	36.7	36.8	37.0
178-182	36.3	36.5	36.6	36.8	36.9	37.1	37.2	37.4	37.5
183-187	36.8	37.0	37.1	37.3	37.4	37.6	37.8	37.9	38.1
188-192	37.3	37.5	37.6	37.8	37.9	38.1	38.2	38.4	38.5
193-197	37.8	38.0	38.1	38.3	38.4	38.6	38.7	38.9	39.0
198-202	38.2	38.4	38.5	38.7	38.8	39.0	39.1	39.3	39.5
203-207	38.7	38.8	39.0	39.1	39.3	39.4	39.6	39.7	39.9
208-212	39.0	39.2	39.3	39.5	39.6	39.8	40.0	40.1	40.3

[1]Skinfolds = chest, thigh, suprailium, abdomen, triceps, and subscapula.
From M.L. Pollock and A.S. Jackson with permission from personal communication.

Table 5 Relative Body Fat From the Sum of Six Skinfolds[1] in Adult Men Under 40 Years of Age (in mm)

Sum of 6 Skinfolds	Age to Last Year							
	Under 19	20 to 22	23 to 25	26 to 28	29 to 31	32 to 34	35 to 37	38 to 40
17- 23	.9	1.3	1.7	2.1	2.5	2.9	3.3	3.7
24- 30	2.3	2.7	3.1	3.5	3.9	4.3	4.7	5.1
31- 37	3.7	4.1	4.5	4.9	5.3	5.7	6.1	6.5
38- 44	5.1	5.5	5.9	6.3	6.7	7.1	7.5	7.9
45- 51	6.4	6.8	7.2	7.6	8.0	8.4	8.8	9.2
52- 58	7.7	8.1	8.5	8.9	9.3	9.7	10.1	10.5
59- 65	9.0	9.4	9.8	10.2	10.6	11.0	11.4	11.8
66- 72	10.2	10.6	11.0	11.4	11.8	12.2	12.6	13.0
73- 79	11.5	11.9	12.3	12.7	13.1	13.5	13.9	14.3
80- 86	12.7	13.1	13.5	13.9	14.3	14.7	15.1	15.5
87- 93	13.8	14.2	14.6	15.0	15.4	15.8	16.2	16.6
94-100	15.0	15.4	15.8	16.2	16.6	17.0	17.4	17.8
101-107	16.1	16.5	16.9	17.3	17.7	18.1	18.5	18.9
108-114	17.1	17.5	17.9	18.3	18.7	19.1	19.5	19.9
115-121	18.2	18.6	19.0	19.4	19.8	20.2	20.6	21.0
122-128	19.2	19.6	20.0	20.4	20.8	21.2	21.6	22.0
129-135	20.2	20.6	21.0	21.4	21.8	22.2	22.6	23.0
136-142	21.2	21.6	22.0	22.4	22.8	23.2	23.6	24.0
143-149	22.1	22.5	22.9	23.3	23.7	24.1	24.5	24.9
150-156	23.0	23.4	23.8	24.2	24.6	25.0	25.4	25.8

(Cont.)

Table 5 (Cont.)

157-163	23.9	24.3	24.7	25.1	25.5	25.9	26.3	26.7
164-170	24.8	25.2	25.6	26.0	26.4	26.8	27.2	27.6
171-177	25.6	26.0	26.4	26.8	27.2	27.6	28.0	28.4
178-184	26.4	26.8	27.2	27.6	28.0	28.4	28.8	29.2
185-191	27.1	27.5	27.9	28.3	28.7	29.1	29.5	29.9
192-198	27.9	28.3	28.7	29.1	29.5	29.9	30.3	30.7
199-205	28.6	29.0	29.4	29.8	30.2	30.6	31.0	31.4
206-212	29.3	29.7	30.1	30.5	30.9	31.3	31.7	32.1
213-219	29.9	30.3	30.7	31.1	31.5	31.9	32.3	32.7
220-226	30.6	31.0	31.4	31.8	32.2	32.6	33.0	33.4
227-233	31.2	31.6	32.0	32.4	32.8	33.2	33.6	34.0
234-240	31.7	32.1	32.5	32.9	33.3	33.7	34.1	34.5
241-247	32.3	32.7	33.1	33.5	33.9	34.3	34.7	35.1
248-254	32.8	33.2	33.6	34.0	34.4	34.8	35.2	35.6
255-261	33.3	33.7	34.1	34.5	34.9	35.3	35.7	36.1
262-268	33.7	34.1	34.5	34.9	35.3	35.7	36.1	36.5
269-275	34.1	34.5	34.9	35.3	35.7	36.1	36.5	36.9
276-282	34.5	34.9	35.3	35.7	36.1	36.5	36.9	37.3
283-289	34.9	35.3	35.7	36.1	36.5	36.9	37.3	37.7
290-296	35.2	35.6	36.0	36.4	36.8	37.2	37.6	38.0

¹Skinfolds = chest, thigh, suprailium, abdomen, triceps, and subscapula.
From M.L. Pollock and A.S. Jackson with permission from personal communication.

Table 6 Relative Body Fat From the Sum of Six Skinfolds[1] in Adult Men 40 Years of Age and Older (in mm)

Sum of 6 Skinfolds	Age to Last Year							
	41 to 43	44 to 46	47 to 49	50 to 52	53 to 55	56 to 58	59 to 61	62 and older
17- 23	4.1	4.5	4.9	5.3	5.7	6.1	6.5	6.9
24- 30	5.5	5.9	6.3	6.7	7.1	7.5	7.9	8.3
31- 37	6.9	7.3	7.7	8.1	8.5	8.9	9.3	9.7
38- 44	8.3	8.7	9.1	9.5	9.9	10.3	10.7	11.1
45- 51	9.6	10.0	10.4	10.8	11.2	11.6	12.0	12.4
52- 58	10.9	11.3	11.7	12.1	12.5	12.9	13.3	13.7
59- 65	12.2	12.6	13.0	13.4	13.8	14.2	14.6	15.0
66- 72	13.4	13.8	14.2	14.6	15.0	15.4	15.8	16.2
73- 79	14.7	15.1	15.5	15.9	16.3	16.7	17.1	17.5
80- 86	15.9	16.3	16.7	17.1	17.5	17.9	18.3	18.7
87- 93	17.0	17.4	17.8	18.2	18.6	19.0	19.4	19.8
94-100	18.2	18.6	19.0	19.4	19.8	20.2	20.6	21.0
101-107	19.3	19.7	20.1	20.5	20.9	21.3	21.7	22.1
108-114	20.3	20.7	21.1	21.5	21.9	22.3	22.7	23.1
115-121	21.4	21.8	22.2	22.6	23.0	23.4	23.8	24.2
122-128	22.4	22.8	23.2	23.6	24.0	24.4	24.8	25.2
129-135	23.4	23.8	24.2	24.6	25.0	25.4	25.8	26.2
136-142	24.4	24.8	25.2	25.6	26.0	26.4	26.8	27.2
143-149	25.3	25.7	26.1	26.5	26.9	27.3	27.7	28.1
150-156	26.2	26.6	27.0	27.4	27.8	28.2	28.6	29.0

(Cont.)

Table 6 (Cont.)

157-163	27.1	27.5	27.9	28.3	28.7	29.1	29.5	29.9
164-170	28.0	28.4	28.8	29.2	29.6	30.0	30.4	30.8
171-177	28.8	29.2	29.6	30.0	30.4	30.8	31.2	31.6
178-184	29.6	30.0	30.4	30.8	31.2	31.6	32.0	32.4
185-191	30.3	30.7	31.1	31.5	31.9	32.3	32.7	33.1
192-198	31.1	31.5	31.9	32.3	32.7	33.1	33.5	33.9
199-205	31.8	32.2	32.6	33.0	33.4	33.8	34.2	34.6
206-212	32.5	32.9	33.3	33.7	34.1	34.5	34.9	35.3
213-219	33.1	33.5	33.9	34.3	34.7	35.1	35.5	35.9
220-226	33.8	34.2	34.6	35.0	35.4	35.8	36.2	36.6
227-233	34.4	34.8	35.2	35.6	36.0	36.4	36.8	37.2
234-240	34.9	35.3	35.7	36.1	36.5	36.9	37.3	37.7
241-247	35.5	35.9	36.3	36.7	37.1	37.5	37.9	38.3
248-254	36.0	36.4	36.8	37.2	37.6	38.0	38.4	38.8
255-261	36.5	36.9	37.3	37.7	38.1	38.5	38.9	39.3
262-268	36.9	37.3	37.7	38.1	38.5	38.9	39.3	39.7
269-275	37.3	37.7	38.1	38.5	38.9	39.3	39.7	40.1
276-282	37.7	38.1	38.5	38.9	39.3	39.7	40.1	40.5
283-289	38.1	38.5	38.9	39.3	39.7	40.1	40.5	40.9
290-296	38.4	38.8	39.2	39.6	40.0	40.4	40.8	41.2

[1]Skinfolds = chest, thigh, suprailium, abdomen, triceps, and subscapula.

From M.L. Pollock and A.S. Jackson with permission from personal communication.

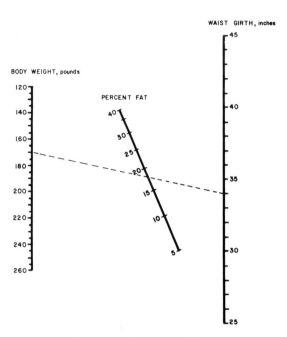

Figure 13   Estimation of relative fat in men from body weight and abdominal or waist circumference

relative body fat from Figure 13. Using a straight-edged device such as a ruler, line up your waist circumference or girth with your body weight, and your relative body fat is that point where the straight edge crosses the percent fat line. The illustration in Figure 13 demonstrates this calculation. With a body weight of 170 pounds and a waist circumference of 34 inches, the percent fat is estimated to be 18.0%. For women, the circumference of the hips is measured at its widest point and the subsequent measurement is used with height to estimate body fat (Figure 14).

How prevalent is the problem of obesity? Unfortunately, few studies have actually measured or estimated body fat; therefore, little data is available on the actual percentage of the American population that would meet the above definition of obesity. According to Dr. George Bray (1979), the percentage of men that are greater than 20% above their desirable weight varies from a low of 7.4% in 20 to 24 year olds, up to 17.0% in 35 to 44 year olds. For women, those who are greater

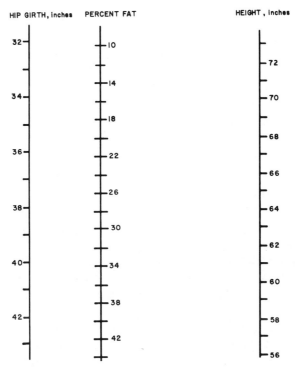

Figure 14   Estimation of relative fat in women from height and hip circumference

than 20% above their desirable weight vary from 9.6% at 20 to 24 years of age, to 34.7% at 55 to 64 years of age.

In both sexes, beyond the age of 25 years, the average individual will gain one pound of weight per year. This does not seem like much since your bathroom scales are usually not that accurate, and your body weight will typically fluctuate from 2 to 5 pounds during the course of a normal day. In addition to this weight gain of one pound per year, there is a loss of approximately one half of a pound of lean weight each year resulting from a loss of lean tissue, primarily muscle and bone. Once the adult reduces his or her basic level of exercise, there will be a decrease in lean tissue, similar to that seen when a broken arm or leg is placed in a cast. With a *net* gain of one pound of weight per year, but a loss of a half of a pound of lean weight per year, this indicates that the average American is accumulating 1½ pounds of fat per year, or 45 pounds of *extra* fat in 30 years, by the age of 55 years. No wonder the average middle-aged American comes home tired at night after a sedentary day's work at the office.

Bruce Hannon and Timothy Lohman (1978) calculated the fossil fuel energy that would be required to supply the extra food calories just to maintain this excess body fat of the total American population. They estimated that there were 377 million kilograms of excess fat in men and 667 million kilograms of excess fat in women, yielding a total of over one billion kilograms or 2.3 billion pounds of excess fat. The actual energy saved by dieting to reach optimal weight and the savings in energy resulting from a lowered food intake to support the optimal body weight, would be more than sufficient to supply the annual residential electrical demands of Boston, Chicago, San Francisco, and Washington, D.C. When expressed in these terms, one can only begin to grasp the significance and magnitude of the problems associated with an obese society.

What is the basic cause of obesity? Over the years, the general population has been led to believe that obesity is the result of gluttony on the one hand, or glandular malfunction on the other. In the last instance, the responsibility is taken away from the individual and the obese condition is blamed on factors beyond the control of the individual. It is now recognized that obesity has many origins—including heredity, early over-nutrition, physical inactivity, social factors, psychological factors, and endocrine and rare syndromes. Of these factors, physical inactivity appears to be one of the most important for several reasons. First, with physical activity you have an additional expenditure of calories. Second, the regulation of appetite and food intake appears to be dependent on certain levels of physical activity. Without adequate activity, the body seems to lose the ability to fine tune the appetite, and extra, unneeded calories are consumed.

What are the ultimate consequences of obesity? The obese individual is at an increased risk for a number of serious medical problems. While hypertension and diabetes are most closely associated with obesity, obesity has also been related to an increased risk for coronary artery disease, venous thrombosis, thrombophlebitis, elevated blood fats, high uric acid levels in the blood (possibly leading to gout), gastrointestinal disorders, respiratory disorders, kidney disease, and gallbladder disease. The obese individual is also at an increased risk for arthritis, surgery, accidents of all types, and, finally, the obese individual often suffers from discrimination, emotional disorders, and restricted life-styles.

Anxiety and Depression

Anxiety and depression are two undesirable psychological states that have reached pandemic proportions in the United States in recent years. Emotional disturbance may be the cause of more marital, professional, and social distress than most organic diseases combined. Anxiety can be defined as a vague feeling of nervousness, apprehension, and uncertainty, and is similar to the feelings associated with a specific cause or threat, but can produce confusion, and distorted perceptions of time and space, and distortion of motivation and meanings of events. It can hinder learning and normal mental processes through lowering of concentration, impairing memory, and decreasing the ability to relate one item to another. Depression is characterized by a sense of hopelessness, self-depreciation, bitterness, regret, and a slowing of emotional responses as well as mental and body functioning. It has been estimated that over 50% of all patients hospitalized with emotional illness have been diagnosed as suffering from various depression disorders.

The causes of anxiety and depression are numerous and often times vague. The physical fitness levels of individuals with emotional or mental disorders is typically low. Whether this is a possible cause or a consequence of the disorder has not been well established. Anxiety and depression are generally of a fairly mild nature with few consequences if treated early. Left untreated, however, the individual can develop serious physiological disorders which can result in complete incapacitation, or even death.

Lower Back Pain, Arthritis, and Osteoporosis

Problems related to lower back pain constitute one of the most frequent medical complaints faced by physicians. It is estimated that 20% to 40% of our adult population have had in the past, or presently have, acute or chronic back pain. It has long been established that muscle weakness and poor flexibility contribute to lower back pain. As early as the mid-1940s clinics were set up to study the possible causes of lower back pain. Of those patients who had chronic back problems, nearly 80% exhibited muscle weakness or poor flexibility, and had no specific disease, lesion, or other medical anomaly that could account for their back problems. Tension and lack of physical activity were major contributing factors in most of these cases. It appears that *exercise has a protective value in the prevention of back pain, directly by keeping posture muscles flexible and strong, and indirectly by its natural tranquilizing effect, controlling nervous tension.*

Arthritis, or "rheumatism," is a disease of the joints characterized by pain and stiffness, and is sometimes crippling. Approximately 12 million to 15 million Americans suffer from the disease. Essentially, there are two different types of arthritis: *rheumatoid arthritis*, and *osteoarthritis*. Rheumatoid arthritis is of unknown origin but can strike early in life and progress rapidly to deformed joints and general crippling. Osteoarthritis is far more common, and appears to be a part of the normal aging process. As one grows older, the joints, like other parts of the body, deteriorate from constant use, or from previous injury. By the age of 60 years, from 80% to 90% of the population have some deterioration of the weight-bearing joints. When the deterioration progresses to the point where movement of these joints becomes painful or difficult, this is then referred to as osteoarthritis. Anything that increases ordinary stress and strain on the joints may bring on osteoarthritis, including overweight, poor posture, and occupations requiring continual use of the joints under conditions of dampness and cold.

There is an associated problem which is related to osteo-arthritis, and that is the fact that there is a general reduction in the mass of bone in the body as one reaches 50 to 60 years of age. This is the result of a loss in bone mineral, primarily calcium, as well as in the bone matrix, the structural compo-nent of bone which supports the bone mineral. While this has been referred to as adult *osteoporosis*, this is not a totally cor-rect designation. In true osteoporosis, there is a loss only in bone mineral, while the matrix remains intact. The conse-quences of this reduction in bone mass are several:

* The total body height will decrease up to an inch or more
* The bones become weaker, or more brittle, and are much more susceptible to fracture
* Once fractured, the bones heal very slowly
* Because of the extended period of immobilization accom-panying fractures particularly for weight-bearing bones, the individual frequently undergoes considerable deteri-oration of all body systems, with death being a frequent consequence (most often in those over 65 years of age)

The causes of the loss of bone mass are not well under-stood at the present time. Diet, hormonal change, as in menopause, and decreased physical activity are the three fac-tors considered to be the most important potential causes, either singularly or in combination.

Promoting an Active Life-Style— Choice or Necessity?

In the previous chapter, the role of physical inactivity was discussed as it related to the most prevalent of the hypokinetic diseases: coronary artery disease, hypertension, obesity, anxiety and depression, and musculoskeletal diseases and disability. While physical inactivity was strongly linked to each of these diseases, this does not imply that by increasing physical activity you can prevent the disease or undergo successful rehabilitation if the disease is present. The health-related benefits of an active and vigorous life-style are somewhat controversial, or, at best, poorly understood. In this chapter, an attempt will be made to describe the role of increased physical activity on each of the hypokinetic diseases defined and discussed previously. Only then can you make a decision as to whether promoting an active life-style is a choice or a necessity.

Coronary Artery Disease—
What Does the Research Have to Say?

Physical inactivity has been listed as a risk factor for coronary artery disease. There are still some researchers and clinicians, however, who seriously question the need for exercise in the prevention of this disease. What does the available research have to offer with respect to linking physical activity to the prevention of heart attacks?

Most of the original research on exercise and heart disease involved observing in large populations the differences in the rate of heart attack and death from heart attack, comparing "sedentary" and "active" groups. It must be mentioned that these types of studies do not necessarily demonstrate absolute cause-effect relationships. However, in over thirty studies, only three failed to confirm that those who were sedentary in their occupation were at a higher risk than those who were active. Again, however, the problems associated with such an approach are many. What about those individuals who are totally sedentary in their occupations, yet may be quite active in their leisure time? They would traditionally be classified as sedentary, yet they may be getting far more exercise and activity than the individual in the active occupation who is relatively sedentary once he or she has left his or her job.

Researchers have gone on to compare groups of people according to how active they are in their leisure time. These studies strongly support the recurring finding that the sedentary individual is at a substantially greater risk for the early development of coronary artery disease when compared to the active individual.

Again, since cause-effect cannot be absolutely demonstrated with studies of this nature, it is also necessary to look at alternative ways of demonstrating a link between physical activity and the prevention of coronary artery disease. One approach is to determine the influence of physical activity on the other risk factors for coronary artery disease. In a comprehensive study of approximately 3,000 men, with an average age of 44.6 years, Cooper and his associates (1976) at the Institute of Aerobics Research in Dallas, Texas, reported that those men who had the highest levels of physical fitness had lower resting heart rates, body weights, percent body fats, blood serum levels of cholesterol and triglycerides, glucose, and systolic blood pressures. Thus, the more fit the individual, the lower the risk for coronary artery disease. Similar results were recently reported in women (Gibbons et al., 1983).

While the above studies were of a cross-sectional nature—the subjects were observed only once—longitudinal studies, where individuals are actually placed on exercise programs, and studied before and after, tend to confirm these results. Exercise programs have been shown to reduce blood pressure in those individuals who are classified as hypertensive, to reduce blood serum levels of cholesterol (minimal change) and triglycerides, to reduce stress and anxiety, to reduce relative and absolute body fat, and to help in the management of the diabetic patient. Also, the American Cancer Society and other groups or agencies have used exercise in their programs for smoking control, and have found exercise to be a good substitute therapy.

Direct evidence for the protective role of exercise in the prevention of coronary artery disease has to come from animal models. Early studies were unable to consistently demonstrate significant differences between animals that exercised versus those that remained sedentary. A recent study by Kramsch and his associates (1981) at the Boston University Medical Center has provided the strongest support to date directly linking physical activity with reduced atherosclerosis. Monkeys were placed in three different groups, two groups eating a known atherogenic diet (high in fat), one exercising and the other remaining sedentary, and the third group which remained sedentary and ate a diet of monkey chow which is low in fat. The exercise group had substantially less overall atherosclerotic development, larger hearts, and wider coronary arteries. Figure 15 provides a comparison of the exercising and sedentary groups that consumed the atherogenic diet, illustrating the substantial difference in the left main coronary artery.

Figure 15   Comparison of the left main coronary artery in sedentary (A) versus exercising (B) monkeys. (From Kramsch, D.M., et al., 1981. *New England Journal of Medicine*, **305**, 1483. Reprinted with permission.)

Even though the cross-sectional and longitudinal studies in humans provide valuable insight into the exercise-heart attack relationship, they still do not provide absolute, irrefutable proof that physical activity is important in preventing heart attacks, and in increasing the chances of survival from heart attacks. While considerable evidence is accumulating each day in support of vigorous exercise, it continues to be of an indirect, rather than direct nature. Samuel M. Fox, III, M.D., prominent cardiologist, recognizes the present dilemma and has proposed the following solution (1969). Rather than either accepting or rejecting a theory on the basis of absolute proof or not, he feels it is acceptable to discuss additional levels of acceptance of preventive or therapeutic approaches: (a) proved beyond reasonable doubt; (b) of probable benefit, but not above question; (c) a prudent action—on the basis of a good chance of benefit, and an acceptably low hazard; and (d) promising, but more good data is needed. At the time this article was written, Dr. Fox concluded that it is prudent to include increased habitual physical activity in a program to prevent or manage nonacute coronary heart disease. Some 16 years later, it would seem appropriate to move up one more rung on the ladder and conclude that exercise is of probable benefit, but not above question.

The major reason for taking a more positive stand for exercise has come from a series of studies conducted recently. Prior to the last few years, there was little evidence to support a mechanism by which vigorous physical activity could alter one's risk for heart attack. Now, these recent studies are starting to uncover that possible mechanism. Cholesterol, implicated as a primary risk factor, is a fatty substance which is both manufactured in the liver and consumed in the diet, and that builds up on the inner wall of the arteries, causing a narrowing of the channel through which the blood must flow. Since cholesterol is not soluble in blood, that is, it will always separate out and rise to the top, if it is to be transported in the blood it must be packaged in a form acceptable in the blood. Cholesterol is carried through the blood by a series of molecules called *lipoproteins*. There are four major lipoproteins:

- The *chylomicrons* are the largest and the lightest lipoproteins, consisting of approximately 80% to 95% triglyceride, 2% to 7% cholesterol, and the remainder is phospholipid and protein.
- *Very low density lipoproteins* (VLDL) are the next largest and lightest lipoproteins, and are composed of approximately 15% cholesterol, 60% triglyceride, with the remainder phospholipid and protein.
- *Low density lipoproteins* (LDL) are a smaller but more dense lipoprotein which are composed of nearly 50%

cholesterol, 5% to 10% triglyceride, and a balance of phospholipid and protein.

- *High density lipoproteins* (HDL) are the smallest and most dense of the lipoproteins and contain approximately 20% cholesterol, 5% triglyceride, and a balance of phospholipid and protein.

Of what significance is the above to coronary artery disease, and specifically to the role of exercise in this disease? Recent studies have found that those individuals with very low levels of HDL and high levels of LDL are at an extremely high risk for heart attack. In fact, high LDL levels may be the single most important risk factor for predicting coronary artery disease. Conversely, high HDL levels appear to provide a degree of protection from coronary artery disease. Thus, one can have normal, or even relatively high, total cholesterol levels, but if it is in the form of HDL cholesterol, it will be a positive, not a negative risk factor.

To date, there have been only five ways identified to alter HDL cholesterol levels: hormones (birth control pills), cessation of smoking, diet, moderate intake of alcohol, and vigorous, endurance exercise. It appears that exercise may exert the greatest influence on elevating HDL cholesterol levels, thus providing possible protection from heart attack. How does HDL cholesterol provide protection? It is presently thought that HDL affixes itself to the arterial wall and actually removes cholesterol from the arterial wall and transports this cholesterol back to the liver where it is either stored or metabolized and excreted. Thus, HDL appears to be a cholesterol scavenger, removing rather than depositing cholesterol in the inside lining of the arterial wall. Dr. Peter Wood and his associates at Stanford University (1979) have pioneered much of this early work relating endurance activity to elevations in HDL cholesterol levels, and to reductions in LDL cholesterol. While there are still many unanswered questions, there is now a strong case that can be made for promoting vigorous exercise of an endurance nature in the prevention of heart attacks.

One word of caution, lest we get too carried away. Direct, absolute proof of the exercise-heart attack prevention link is still missing. We should be wary of enthusiasts who make claims that if one is able to run distances such as a marathon, that virtual immunity from fatal heart attacks is assured. Thomas J. Bassler, M.D., a pathologist and an active marathoner, once stated (1975), "As no cases of fatal athero-sclerosis have been documented in marathon finishers of any age, it follows that such activity confers virtual immunity from fatal heart attacks," and that "immunity to a heart attack coexists with the ability to cover 42 kilometers on foot." Unfortunately, Dr. Bassler's statements were totally conjecture at that time, and were not based on scientific fact. While the motives of individuals who make such claims are probably pure and are an attempt to promote an active life-style in a sedentary population, such claims only serve to confuse the basic issues, and, in some cases, actually work to discourage the sedentary individual from exercising, since it can be difficult even to visualize the walking of a mile. Jogging or running 26.2 miles would seem to be totally impossible.

Hypertension

The role of exercise in treating hypertension is somewhat better understood. Many of the early studies observing the influence of regular endurance exercise on resting blood pressure found little or no change in either systolic or diastolic blood pressure following weeks to months of vigorous exercise. It was only later that it became apparent that most of these studies were conducted on populations that essentially had normal blood pressure. Thus, it wasn't surprising to find normal blood pressures staying approximately the same. When studies were conducted on individuals who were truly hypertensive (elevated systolic and/or diastolic pressure) they found that blood pressures were lowered toward normal levels with endurance training. It should be mentioned, however, that the best control of hypertension is through a combination of diet, restricting salt intake as well as total calories, weight reduction, and exercise. If, after a period of 6 months to a year, the blood pressure levels have not dropped to satisfactory levels, it may be necessary for the patient's physician to prescribe anti-hypertension medication. In all cases, however, the total management of the patient should be under the direct supervision of his or her personal physician.

Obesity

It is often thought that exercise is a very inefficient method of weight loss and weight control. A common belief is that it takes far too much exercise to lose a single pound of fat (you must chop wood for 7 hours, walk 35 miles, or climb a 10-foot staircase 1,000 times). Another common argument states that exercise only serves to increase the appetite, and this increase in calories consumed will be equal to or even exceed the number of calories used to perform the exercise.

Both of these arguments are misleading and erroneous. In fact, research has proven that exercise may be one of the more efficient ways to lose weight and keep the weight off. As we stated earlier, inactivity is a major cause of obesity in the United States. Thus, exercise must also be recognized as a significant factor in any program of weight reduction or control. Keep the following factors in mind when evaluating an exercise program for weight loss, or more specifically, fat loss.

First, it requires the expenditure of approximately 3,500 calories to lose a pound of fat. This 3,500 calorie deficit can be accomplished in one of three ways: dieting, exercise, or a combination of diet and exercise. By taking one buttered slice of bread out of the diet each day (approximately 100 calories), the individual would lose one pound of fat in 35 days, providing everything else remained constant. Likewise, one pound of fat could be lost in 35 days by walking or jogging one mile each day (approximately 100 calories expended per mile), again assuming all other factors remained constant. By combining this modest decrease in food intake and increase in activity level, it would be possible to lose the same pound of fat in only half of that time, 17½ days. One could speed up the process of fat loss considerably. As an example, by walking 5 miles a day (500 calories) and decreasing food intake by 500 calories per day, it would be possible to have a total caloric deficit of 1,000 calories per day, which would allow the loss of 1 pound of fat every 3½ days, or 2 pounds of fat loss per week.

Unrealistic Expectations

However, the above approach doesn't appeal to the general American population, for we are a society that is geared for the immediate—the "now generation." We are accustomed to having whatever we want, whenever we want it. This same philosophy applies to almost all walks of life. The young woman who is 30 pounds above desirable weight, and who is invited to the big dance of the year which is just 1 month away, decides it is time to lose that weight so she will have a desirable appearance on the night of the dance. The weight loss goal of 30 pounds is admirable, but the time sequence of 1 pound weight loss per day is totally unreasonable. The "paunchy" middle-aged male who is due to return for a reunion of his high school graduating class is confronted with the problem of being 50 pounds overweight, and with the reunion only 6 weeks away, he decides that it is time to get back into shape. Again, this goal is noble but the expectation is unrealistic. The eating and exercise habits (or lack of) that resulted in the person's current weight took time, usually years, to develop. It only makes sense that it could take months or even years to change those habits significantly.

The American population spends billions of dollars each year in combating the "battle of the bulge," only in most instances to face a losing battle. Weight which is rapidly lost is frequently regained even more rapidly. As new diets are introduced this cycle repeats itself. Dr. Jean Mayer, president of Tufts University, and world-famous nutritionist, formerly of Harvard University, has coined the term to describe this phenomenon as the "rhythm method" of girth control. Such repetitive patterns of weight loss and weight gain are psychologically destructive to the individual and can also have serious medical implications over time.

What is the basic cause of these weight control failures, and how does this relate to the use of exercise in weight reduction and weight control? The major cause of failure in most weight loss programs relates to the urgency factor; once the decision is made to lose the weight, the desired weight loss must be accomplished immediately. This frequently leads to a search for the latest fad diet. Unfortunately, nutrition is an area which has spawned many self-proclaimed experts, so if one has the appropriate credentials, such as an MD or PhD degree, this allows that individual license to develop the next wonder diet in which it is claimed to be possible to lose 5 to 10 pounds per week with only "minor" modifications in one's life-style. In the past, we have heard that "calories don't count," and that you can eat as much as you want, providing you eat only certain foods. Most of us even know of friends or relatives who have lost 5 to 10 pounds per week using one of the modern miracle diets. Yet, the results remain basically the same, quick weight loss and rapid weight gain once the dieting period has ended.

Rapid-Weight-Loss Diets

Rapid-weight-loss strategies typically do not work for very simple reasons. Using 3,500 calories as the equivalent of 1 pound of fat loss, it would be possible to lose no more than 1 pound of weight per day if one were to totally abstain from food intake, and expend 3,500 calories every 24 hours. The average adult male and female who engage in moderate levels of activity need approximately 2,800 and 2,000 calories, respectively, to maintain their body weight; that is, such a diet over an extended period of time will result in neither a weight loss nor a weight gain. Thus, to attain a 1 pound per day loss of fat, the average male would have to use 700 additional calories in exercise (equivalent to walking or jogging 7 miles) as well as to refrain from eating. The average female would have to expend an extra 1,500 calories in exercise (walking or jogging 15 miles) in addition to abstaining from food. It is obvious that these are totally unrealistic approaches to weight loss, yet how can we explain the 5 to 10 pound weight losses some individuals experience in a 1-week period of time?

Most rapid-weight-loss diets have one thing in common— they allow only a modest intake of carbohydrates. Carbohydrates constitute approximately 60% of the normal mixed diet. When carbohydrate intake is lowered to levels of 10% or less of the total food intake, combined with a reduction in total food intake, the body starts to utilize its own carbohydrate stores in the liver and muscles. When you store a gram of carbohydrate in the liver or muscles, you store along with it approximately 3 grams of water. When you use a gram of carbohydrate from the body stores, you will lose 3 grams of water. Thus, as the body stores of carbohydrate are being reduced as a result of a low-calorie diet deficient in carbohydrate, there will be a substantial loss of body water. Also, additional water is lost as a result of the greater utilization of fat, which results in an increased production of *ketone bodies*, which are by-products of fat metabolism. *Ketosis*, or an elevation of ketone bodies in the blood, frequently results and is characterized by a distinct acetone odor on the breath. The ketone bodies will spill into the urine; thus, many of these diets encourage self-administered, periodic testing of the urine with ketone sticks to keep this condition under control. Prolonged periods of ketosis can have substantial detrimental effects on the body. The combined effects of ketosis and utilization of the body's carbohydrate stores results in a substantial loss of water. Thus, the large losses of weight that occur within the first few weeks of dieting are essentially losses of body fluids, not body fat. In fact, several studies have demonstrated that from 60% to 70% of this weight loss during the initial 10 to 14 days on these diets is from the lean body tissue, which includes the body fluids.

For the average female, it is literally impossible to lose more than 3 pounds of fat per week, even under the most extreme conditions. If the average female who normally consumes 2,000 calories to maintain body weight were to fast for a period of 1 week, which is not a recommended procedure, she would theoretically lose the fat equivalent of 2,000 calories per day, or nearly 0.6 of a pound per day (2,000 cal. ÷ 3,500 cal./lb. = 0.57 lb.). *However, when you reduce your food intake to starvation or near-starvation levels, the body reduces its energy needs by 25% to 30%*. Thus, where the body was requiring 2,000 calories per day with normal food intake, it requires substantially less when it is under the stress of inadequate food intake, that is, 1,400 to 1,500 calories. The equivalent amount of fat lost per day is reduced accordingly to approximately 0.4 of a pound, or 2.8 pounds per week with total starvation.

Referring back to the previous discussion, it was shown that by combining diet and exercise, it was possible to achieve a deficit of 1,000 calories per day, which is equivalent to approximately 2 pounds of fat loss per week. While this may appear to be the slow approach to weight loss, it is the most sensible approach. Losses of lean tissue are minimal, and research evidence indicates that the losses are more likely to be of a permanent nature. The success or failure of any weight loss program should be measured only after a period of several years have passed from the time that the desired weight was attained. If the weight loss has been maintained, then the program can be considered a success.

The reason the rapid-weight-loss programs so often result in failure is the fact that once a desired weight is achieved, the individual typically will return to a normal diet, which is high in carbohydrates. The water which was lost during the dieting period is quickly regained, often in a matter of only a few days. Thus, the individual's weight literally jumps back to its previous level, and the diet is considered a failure. The goal should be the development of new diet and exercise habits that will result both in the desired weight loss *and* the long-term maintenance of lower weight. "Fad" diets and "crash" exercise programs will not do this.

Exercise and Weight Loss

Exercise is, therefore, an essential part of any sound weight reduction and weight control program. While it does take considerable activity to achieve a significant weight loss, chances are it will be a permanent weight loss. Many research studies have confirmed the fact that it is possible to lose approximately a quarter of a pound of fat per week from an exercise program that requires no more than 3 days per week, 30 minutes per day. This would be approximately the equivalent of walking or jogging 9 miles per week. While this doesn't seem like much, this rate of fat loss would result in a total loss in 1 year of 13 pounds, and this is from exercise alone. These results can be even more substantial when *moderate* dieting is included.

Doesn't exercise increase the appetite so you take in more food? Several studies on humans as well as animals have shown that moderate levels of activity even tend to decrease one's appetite for up to several hours after exercising. Individuals who have started exercise programs, such as jogging, find that if they exercise just prior to their biggest meal, which is typically dinner, they will not eat as much—the appetite is just not there. Increasing evidence is accumulating which is suggesting that the body must have a certain basic level of exercise before it is able to regulate appetite, and thus food intake, to match the energy expenditure. If activity levels drop below this basic level, the body loses its ability to "fine-tune" the appetite, with a resulting increase in food consumption above that which is needed. This inability to fine-tune may result in only a seemingly small imbalance of 10 calories per day (approximately one potato chip), but over a period of 1 year this adds an excess of 3,600 calories per year, or the equivalent of an added pound of fat.

When using an exercise program to complement dieting in weight reduction, it is important to remember that as we get older we lose lean tissue, primarily muscle and bone mass, as we discussed earlier. This is the result of an increasingly sedentary life-style. However, when one starts to exercise, this process reverses itself and the body tends to gain lean weight. Thus, it is not uncommon to find little or no change in the scale or total body weight over the first few weeks to months that the individual is on the program. This is normal and should be expected. Fat weight is being lost, but lean weight is being gained in approximately the same amount. This could leave you with the impression that the program is a failure, since there is little or no change in scale weight, yet fat is being lost. Do not use the scale as a means of judging progress over the first few months. A far better indicator of those changes is the way clothes fit, for there is a redistribution of the weight, leading to a much more desirable figure or physique. The increase in lean body weight will tend to level off after the first few months in the program. At this point, there will be a detectable reduction in body weight as fat weight will continue to decrease.

Lastly, in addition to a formal exercise program, attempting to be more active in all aspects of your life can also result in substantial dividends. Even small increases or decreases in activity level can have a significant influence on our body fat levels. Most of us spend at least 8 hours per day at work, or approximately 50% of our waking hours, or a third to a fourth of our lives. Thus, any extra activity that can be structured into the work day on a regular basis will have an influence over an extended period of time. Taking stairs instead of elevators or escalators, parking two or three blocks farther from work than where you normally park, or just performing your daily activities in a more active manner will all work toward the common goal of increasing caloric expenditure and decreasing elevated fat stores to more normal levels. The treatment of obesity is a long-term project, and anyone who wishes to lose even small amounts of weight should project a weight loss goal of no more than 1 or 2 pounds per week, and even this should be done with the approval of a family physician. Better yet, prevention should start early in life, avoiding the need in later life for corrective measures.

Anxiety and Depression

A low physical fitness profile is frequently found in patients with various mental diseases or illnesses. Is there a direct cause-effect relationship, or do these two factors simply coexist, both the result of another factor which has not been identified? If there is a direct cause-effect relationship, which factor is the causative factor? Often, inactivity is the result of the disease itself, as in schizophrenics and other psychotic patients who are characterized by a significant general passivity, impaired mobility, lack of communication, and a tendency to autistic thinking and regression which results in an even greater reduction in physical endurance capacity and muscular strength. Also, in various neurotic states, there is a tendency to avoid physical activity for fear that that activity will precipitate serious medical consequences, for example, fast heart rate leading to a fatal heart attack. In addition, certain drugs used in the treatment of mental disorders have side effects which would tend to reduce normal levels of physical activity. There is little, if any, direct evidence that indicates that reduced levels of physical activity leading to low levels of physical fitness are related to the onset of the various mental diseases. It is quite possible that physical inactivity, per se, is not the specific cause, but creates an environment which increases the likelihood of that individual developing that particular mental or emotional disorder. Additional research will be necessary to determine if exercise or the lack of exercise plays a specific role in either preventing (exercise) or causing (lack of exercise) specific mental diseases. In the meantime, a growing body of knowledge is pointing to the importance of cardiovascular endurance exercises in the treatment of mental disorders.

Many studies report reductions in tension and anxiety with increased activity. Here are some of the findings:

- A significant reduction in muscular tension resulted from increased activity.
- Exercise was more effective in reducing muscular tension than a commonly used tranquilizer.
- Techniques such as progressive relaxation, biofeedback, meditation, and hypnosis all reduce anxiety and tension to an extent similar to that achieved with exercise.
- Exercise must approach 70% to 80% of an individual's capacity to achieve a reduction in anxiety.
- Regular endurance exercise has resulted in decreased depression; running seems to be particularly effective, more so than golf or tennis. Previously depressed subjects experienced significantly increased feelings of cheerfulness, energy and activation after starting a jogging program.

It is a common finding that individuals who are involved in a program of regular physical activity of an endurance nature have an increased sense of well-being. In fact, William Glasser (1976), in his book *Positive Addiction*, has reported that joggers or runners who exercise 30 to 60 minutes per day, 4 days a week or more, frequently become addicted to this routine. If illness, injury, travel, or some other interruption disrupts their exercise routine, these individuals actually go through withdrawal-like symptoms! For the non-exerciser, it is difficult to comprehend how vigorous exercise could provide such pleasure.

It does appear that vigorous physical activity of an endurance nature does promote good mental health, particularly in the areas of anxiety and depression. While many of those studies that have been conducted to date could be criticized for being poorly controlled or improperly designed, the evidence is sufficient to allow one to conclude that a healthy mind is typically found in a healthy body, and that physical activity of an endurance nature will improve the health of the mind as well as the body.

Lower Back Pain, Arthritis, and Osteoporosis

While problems of the lower back are a major medical complaint of a substantial percentage of our adult population, most of these problems, approximately 80%, can be linked to a combination of reduced range of movement in the various joints of the body (inflexibility) and inadequate muscular strength to properly support the structure and weight of the body. Fortunately, these are problems that can be corrected with the appropriate selection of flexibility and strength exercises. In one study, where 233 patients with lower back complaints were followed for a period of approximately 8 years, 82% reported substantial therapeutic improvement following an exercise program which emphasized the development of strength and flexibility. Even patients with osteoarthritic changes greatly increased their functional potential with adequate exercise. The National YMCA instituted a program in over 700 YMCAs around the country for treating back pain due to muscle deficiency which is referred to as "The Y's Way to a Healthy Back." This program emphasizes stretching and strength-type exercise, and has produced excellent improvement in 29%, good improvement in 36%, and fair improvement in 25% of a sample of 421 participants representing 19 YMCAs.

With respect to lower back problems, this appears to be one area where improvement can occur within a relatively short period of time, providing the condition is the result of inflexibility and weak musculature. Simple stretching and strengthening exercises done for 10 to 20 minutes per day can bring almost immediate relief, but the program must be maintained indefinitely or the problem will typically recur.

With respect to those changes in bone which result from aging, for example, osteoarthritis and osteoporosis, regular exercise has been shown to provide limited if not substantial alterations in bone metabolism which appear to slow down the general progressive deterioration that results with aging. A study involving women with an average age of 82 years showed increases of 4.2% in bone mineral when these women exercised at light to moderate levels, 30 minutes a day, 3 days a week, for 36 months. A sedentary control group experienced a 2.5% decrease over the same time span. It is known from a number of studies conducted on farm animals and humans that enforced periods of inactivity can lead to substantial decreases in bone mineral. This was a major concern when NASA was initially considering extended periods of space flight. Results from the early space flights indicated the astronauts were experiencing rather substantial losses in bone mineral following these periods of weightlessness in a confined environment. The extended missions, including SkyLab, made provisions for exercise on board the space vehicle or laboratory, to minimize changes in bone mineral as well as to reduce the possibility of general cardiovascular deconditioning. Bone apparently needs the stress of bearing the body weight in order to be maintained at optimal efficiency.

Preventive Medicine—A Total Approach to Health Care

From the preceding, it would appear wise if not essential, that exercise become an important addition to the life-style of the typically inactive person, whether a young child or a senior citizen. For those who have established good exercise habits and enjoy what they are doing, they should be encouraged to continue, for exercise is a lifetime pursuit. One cannot engage in an exercise program for a period of weeks, months, or even years, and then stop to assume a sedentary life-style, expecting to live on the residual benefits of the previous activity. Many alterations in bodily function occur with physical activity that are beneficial to the total health of the individual. However, these benefits are quickly lost when activity is discontinued or interrupted for an extended period of time. For those individuals who have been sedentary, activity should be gradually included as a part of their daily schedule or routine. While it may seem impossible to crowd even more into an already overcommitted schedule, and many may feel that they cannot justify this additional commitment as an efficient use of their time, the ultimate benefits to be derived from a regular program of vigorous activity may indeed make the exercise period the cornerstone of each day's activities. Factors such as improved self-image, with the accompanying improvement in self-confidence, the need for less sleep, the release of anxiety and tension, in addition to the general sense of well-being that accompanies a regular program of vigorous activity, will actually provide dividends in time that will far outweigh the minimal time investment required on a daily basis. In short, physical activity increases the overall efficiency of the body to a level where optimal function is achieved in nearly all aspects of life.

However, exercise is only one aspect of a total approach to health care. There are many other factors which, when combined, provide for optimal health, and contribute to *preventive medicine*. Over the past few years, the concept of preventive medicine has undergone a rather radical and important change. In the past, preventive medicine was essentially limited in concept to such essential practices as providing inoculations to prevent specific diseases, and the treatment of water and sewage to prevent the spread of various diseases. Recently, it has become increasingly apparent that the responsibility for health care can also be shared by the individual. There is much every person can do to promote health and reduce the risk of disease and disability in their own lives. In addition to increasing physical activity, individuals can alter their diets, decrease or stop smoking, reduce alcohol intake to more reasonable levels, allow sufficient time for sleep, and reduce those factors in their present life-style which contribute to increased levels of emotional stress and anxiety.

Often, a person recognizes a need for a drastic change in his or her life-style, either as a result of an existing health problem, or the feeling and fear of impending sickness. This is frequently the major motivator which results in these individuals undertaking an exercise program. While this in itself is not bad, all too often these same individuals have additional unhealthy habits which should be changed, but they feel that exercise alone will provide them with an instant cure, allowing them to continue their other bad habits. This is not an uncommon pattern for those who have had heart attacks and are heavy smokers. These individuals will frequently join a cardiac rehabilitation program where they can start the process of physical reconditioning with the hope and expectation that this alone will resolve their heart problem, allowing them to continue smoking. To concentrate on only one risk factor to the exclusion of others which may be present is unwise. A person's total life-style must be evaluated, and attention should be given to all factors which indicate a risk for any preventable disease.

An additional factor of importance to the total concept of preventive medicine is the periodic medical examination. It has been estimated that the risk of death from various preventable diseases can be reduced by 50% or more simply by having an annual or semi-annual medical examination. Properly conducted, the medical examination can identify various diseases in their early stages, providing a much better chance for total cure or control of the disease. Early detection procedures have been identified for coronary heart disease, hypertension, various forms of cancer, diabetes, and various respiratory diseases, among others. Too often, a disease is detected only in its terminal stages, and this reduces considerably the chances for survival. While no one wants to be told he or she has a serious disease or medical problem, it is far better to have advanced warning where corrective procedures can be instituted early in the course of the disease, thereby increasing the chances of survival and/or recovery to full health and a productive life.

At what age should one start having periodic medical examinations, and how frequently should these be administered? Undoubtedly, the best time to start with a comprehensive medical examination is early in life when health is at its peak. A comprehensive medical examination at age 20 to 25 years provides an excellent base-line examination which can serve as a reference for examinations later in life when health is starting to fail. There is considerable individual variation of normal values for just about all parameters measured in a medical examination. When an individual develops a specific disease or medical problem and a medical profile is measured against the population norms, it may be difficult, if not impossible, to establish an accurate diagnosis since the individual's values for any one test may fall within the rather broad range of values considered normal for that test, while being well out of line for what is normal for that individual. The base-line examination, taken at an early age during a period of optimal health, will provide an invaluable reference throughout life, enabling the comparison of all subsequent examinations to determine when any one test starts to vary from normal, based on that individual's normal range of variation for that specific test. A comprehensive medical examination every 2 or 3 years is recommended for those who have no specific complaints, up to the age of 35 to 45 years of age, at which point an annual examination is recommended. Preventive maintenance has been proven to minimize mechanical failures and to prolong the life of an automobile. A similar program of preventive maintenance is essential for promoting our health and reducing the risk of serious disease and disability.

P   A   R   T

An Exercise Plan for Fitness and Sport

During the past decade a number of advances have been made in the exercise and sport sciences which have had a major influence on the development of safe and sound guidelines for the prescription of exercise. It wasn't too many years ago that exercise programs were initiated with everyone performing the same activity and doing essentially the same sequence at the same intensity of performance. Individuals would line up by the rows to perform in unison an entire series of calisthenic-type exercises, followed by several laps around the gymnasium, an enthusiastic game of volleyball or basketball, several more laps around the gym, and then on to the showers. This was very typical of many of the YMCA, YWCA, or Jewish Community Center programs of the 1950s. At that time, these were considered excellent programs for the development of physical fitness and the promotion of health. Today, the prescription of exercise must be individualized. It is also known that different sports and activities provide widely different benefits. In addition, the benefits of exercise have been proven to vary considerably with the intensity at which the individual plays an activity, in addition to the number of minutes per day and the number of days of the week the individual is involved.

Part II presents a detailed examination of those factors which should be considered when initiating an exercise program. A thorough medical evaluation should precede any formal prescription of exercise. The contents of such an evaluation will be described in addition to outlining those medical problems which would preclude formal exercise under any conditions, or where the risk is sufficiently great to indicate the need for a structured program under the close supervision of a physician. The essential ingredients of a sound, comprehensive exercise prescription are then outlined, followed by a discussion of appropriate warm-up, cool-down, and flexibility exercises; activities to promote cardiorespiratory fitness; training for strength, power, and muscular endurance; and finally the role of sport and recreational activities in the promotion of fitness and sport.

3

C H A P T E R

Medical Examination and Clearance for Exercise

It is relatively uncommon for the average individual to consult a private physician prior to starting an exercise program. However, it is now well documented that a certain percentage of individuals who assume they are healthy, with no apparent disease or risk for disease, will have on closer examination a serious medical problem that will: (a) dictate additional diagnostic procedures and further medical follow-up; (b) place limitations on the exercise prescription, including the possibility of allowing exercise only under the close supervision of a physician or a trained paramedical associate; or (c) preclude the prescription of exercise altogether. The percentage of those who would be identified as having a serious medical problem will vary considerably according to age. Probably fewer than 2% to 5% of those between the ages of 5 and 25 years would fall into this category. However, the older one is, the longer he or she has been sedentary, and the more undesirable health habits he or she has acquired over the years, the greater the risk of falling into this category of having a serious medical problem, or being at a higher risk for a serious medical problem. Many studies have concluded that from 5% to 15% of the normal, presumably healthy adult population will have serious abnormalities in their exercise electrocardiograms which indicate the presence of severe coronary artery disease. In several of these studies, these individuals were found to be "healthy" following a standard physical examination, including a resting electrocardiogram. Their disease was diagnosed only as a result of the exercise electrocardiogram, a test which is not typically a part of a routine physical examination.

From the above, it is suggested that a comprehensive medical evaluation be undertaken prior to initiating any formal program of exercise. This obviously will be more important for those of us 30 years of age and older, but a sound medical evaluation is considered prudent even for the youngster who is just beginning to participate in competitive sports, whether it be Pop Warner Football, Little League Baseball, or junior high school gymnastics. An annual or semi-annual medical evaluation is considered to be a wise investment as a part of a comprehensive program of preventive medicine; thus, a clearance to participate in either sport or fitness activities could be included as a part of this examination at little or no extra cost.

Comprehensive Medical Evaluation

The standard medical examination provided today varies considerably, from a cursory 5-minute assessment of height, weight, blood pressure, and chest sounds, to a comprehensive, multi-phasic evaluation which takes several days to complete. What constitutes an appropriate medical evaluation for clearing individuals for participation in sport or exercise programs? The answer to this question depends entirely on the age of the individual and the activity or sport for which that individual is seeking clearance. The scholastic, collegiate, or professional athlete who is seeking clearance to play football will have a totally different evaluation from the middle-aged adult who is seeking clearance to join the local health club, or who wants to start a jogging program.

Athletic Evaluation

The evaluation for clearing athletes into various sports, while concerned with the general health of the individual, includes as the major component a thorough orthopedic evaluation to identify existing injuries to bones, muscles, ligaments, tendons, and joints, and to evaluate the potential for injury. As an example, a young athlete who is diagnosed as having instability of both knees should be directed out of a high-risk contact sport such as football and encouraged to participate in a nonweight-bearing activity such as swimming or bicycling. Also included in the evaluation of athletes would be a thorough screening for cardiovascular and blood related problems. In the past several years, a number of young and apparently healthy athletes have died either during or following a particularly hard practice or a game. Cardiac arrythmias (irregular heartbeats), myocarditis (infection in the heart muscle), mitral valve prolapse (failure of the mitral valve, allowing blood to flow back into the left atrium on contraction of the left ventricle), congenital heart disease, rheumatic fever, heart attack, and sickle-cell anemia have all been implicated as primary causes of death. Most of these problems are diagnosable; thus, the appropriate cardiovascular screening procedures are essential. Finally, the athletic evaluation should include routine screening of the ears, eyes, urine, and blood. X rays are desirable, but very expensive. They may be required for certain sports, but only recommended for others.

Before leaving this area of athletic evaluations, it is important to recognize that there are a number of physiological changes with endurance training which mimic serious medical problems. One of the classic alterations with endurance training is a substantial reduction in the resting heart rate. Many physicians are greatly concerned when they identify resting heart rates below 60 beats per minute, because it may be an abnormally slow pulse or heartbeat which is the result of disease. In the highly trained endurance athlete, this is a normal response to training and is associated with an elevated stroke volume (volume of blood pumped each beat), thus allowing for a normal cardiac output (volume of blood pumped per minute). Endurance-trained athletes have resting heart rates which are typically below 40 beats per minute, with certain individuals dropping to levels of 30 beats per minute or lower. These unusually low heart rates will frequently lead to arrythmias, where the athlete will sense an early or a late beat, or an extra or a skipped beat. At very slow heart rates, the heart is very susceptible to other areas of the heart taking over the pacemaker activity, since heart tissue has its own natural rate of contraction, totally independent of autonomic nervous system control.

Closely related to the above, many athletes have resting electrocardiograms which are indicative of serious heart diseases. It has only been within the past 10 to 20 years that the medical community has come to recognize these apparent abnormal electrocardiograms as normal in the highly trained athlete. For years, athletes were either sidelined or misdiagnosed as having serious heart disease. Now it is an accepted fact that many of these traditional abnormalities are normal variations for this highly select population of athletes. The "athlete's heart" is also another misclassification as an abnormal heart condition. Electrocardiograms and X rays indicated an enlarged left ventricle in a number of endurance-trained athletes, which in the untrained, nonathlete is a definite indication of heart disease and abnormal heart function. It is now recognized that the increase in the wall thickness and chamber size of the left ventricle is a normal response to both endurance and burst-type activity. This increase in wall thickness allows for a more forceful contraction of the heart, enhancing stroke volume.

Another area in which a medical problem is diagnosed, when, in fact, the "problem" is usually a normal response to chronic endurance training, is the low hematocrit, which is typically associated with anemia. While the hematocrit (ratio of the red blood cells to the total blood volume) is typically low in endurance-trained athletes, either approaching or below values considered indicative of anemia in the normal individual, these athletes will have a total hemoglobin and total number of red blood cells above normal. Anemia is defined as a deficiency in either quantity or quality of blood, with the reduced quality of blood being reflected by either or both a decrease in hemoglobin levels or red blood cells. In the case of the endurance-trained athlete, the quantity as well as the quality of blood are typically well above normal values. The greatly increased plasma volume, however, is expanded to a much greater degree, a liter or more, than the increases in red blood cells and hemoglobin; thus, it appears as if the athlete is anemic, when, in fact, he or she has above-average hemoglobin and red blood cells, which are simply diluted by a greater increase in the fluid portion of the blood.

The above represent only a few of the more common problems where athletes have been misdiagnosed as having a serious disease or a clinical abnormality. In some cases, the failure to recognize the true significance of these apparent problems has resulted in the athlete being disqualified for further competition. A good general rule to follow if a significant medical abnormality is diagnosed is to get a second or third opinion by a physician or physicians who are experienced in working with athletes. Further diagnostic tests can also be administered, in some cases, to determine if there is a significant medical problem that would expose the athlete to a high risk.

Fitness Evaluation

The medical evaluation for clearance into physical fitness programs, as was mentioned earlier, has a totally different focus from the athletic evaluation, although there are many similarities between the two. Typically, the medical evaluation for clearing participants into physical fitness programs is conducted on adults, and, thus, the identification of existing cardiovascular disease, or the risk for subsequent cardiovascular disease, becomes a dominant factor.

What should be included in a standard medical evaluation designed to clear a middle-aged adult into a comprehensive exercise program? First, it is important that the individual's physician have a comprehensive medical history, including the individual's family, as well as a personal medical history. The family history should include incidence of heart disease, stroke, seizures, and disorders of equilibrium in close relatives, with an accurate cause and age at death. The individual's personal medical history should include any history of cardiovascular disease, including heart attacks, angina pectoris, undiagnosed chest pain, hypertension, rheumatic fever, murmurs, and the presence of any factors which place the individual at increased risk for coronary disease; fainting; seizures; or unstable gait. Present medication and treatment, eating habits and diet analysis, smoking history, history of alcohol intake, and present patterns of physical activity should also be noted, along with existing athletic injuries and orthopedic problems.

Once the medical history has been obtained, the physician can start the physical examination, using the medical history as a guide in pinpointing potential problem areas. A family history of heart disease, coupled with the symptom or complaint of chest pains on exertion, leads the physician to suspect underlying coronary artery disease, and the physical examination and diagnostic tests will be oriented in that direction. The general physical examination, however, should include an investigation of bone and joint abnormalities, heart murmurs, cardiac arrythmias, abnormalities in the resting electrocardiogram, blood pressure, the presence of pulmonary emphysema or other chronic lung diseases, and the pulses in both lower extremities.

Other diagnostic tests are highly desirable in order to more completely evaluate the individual's risk for coronary artery disease. A simple blood test can provide information on blood glucose levels (elevated blood glucose levels lead to the suspicion of diabetes, a significant risk factor for coronary artery disease); total cholesterol levels and the levels of high and low density lipoprotein cholesterol; triglyceride levels; and uric acid levels. In addition, it is strongly suggested that anyone who is considered to have a substantial risk for coronary artery disease, or any individual 35 to 40 years of age and over, should have an exercise electrocardiogram. Table 7 provides a greatly simplified procedure for estimating your level of risk for each of the recognized coronary artery disease risk factors.

Table 7 Possible Risk of the Premature Development of Coronary Artery Disease

Risk Factors	Very Low Risk	Low Risk	Average Risk	Moderate Risk	High Risk
PRIMARY					
Blood pressure, mmHg					
Systolic pressure	<110	110-120	121-140	141-160	>160
Diastolic pressure	<60	60-70	71-90	91-105	>105
Cigarettes, per day	none	none	<10	11-30	>30
Blood lipids, mg/100 ml					
Cholesterol					
Total	<180	180-195	196-220	221-260	>260
HDL, males	>64	55-64	45-54	25-44	<25
females	>74	65-74	55-64	35-54	<35
Triglycerides	<80	80-105	106-145	146-190	>190
SECONDARY					
Glucose, mg/100 ml	<80	80-95	96-115	116-135	>135
Body fat, %					
males	<10	10-14	15-20	21-26	>26
females	<15	16-20	21-26	27-33	>33
Stress-tension (subjective)	low	average	moderate	high	very high
Physical activity,[1] minutes	>120	60-120	15-59	<15	none
Exercise electrocardiogram	normal	normal	normal	possibly abnormal	abnormal
Family history[2]	0	0	1	2	>2
Age	<31	31-40	41-50	51-60	>60
Sex		female		male	

[1]Minutes per week exercising at a heart rate in excess of a target rate established by subtracting your age from 220 and multiplying by 0.75 {(220 − age) × 0.75} to be sustained for a minimum of 10 minutes each exercise bout.

[2]Number of blood relatives who had heart attacks prior to age 60 years.

It should be emphasized that this is strictly a guide, and it is based on the best evidence available at this time. It is also important to recognize that all doctors do not agree as to the validity of such a risk evaluation.

The exercise electrocardiogram has become an extremely important diagnostic tool. It was mentioned in the introduction to this chapter that in normal populations who are presumed to be healthy, and have normal resting electrocardiograms, a small but significant number of these individuals will exhibit changes in their electrocardiogram with exercise, which are indicative or suggestive of the presence of coronary artery disease. The estimates vary between 5% and 15%, depending on the sex and age of the individual. It is obviously important to identify those who have these abnormalities, for they can then be referred for further diagnostic evaluation. In some cases, these abnormal responses of the electrocardiogram during exercise are not good predictors of the presence of the disease. These are termed "false positives" on the basis of an abnormal exercise electrocardiogram, but with normal coronary arteries.

Other more involved tests can be used to determine the health of the arteries. The number of false positives, however, is relatively small. Therefore, there is strong support for the use of the exercise electrocardiogram both as a screening test for clearing individuals for participation in exercise programs, and as a diagnostic test to evaluate for the presence or absence of coronary artery disease.

One of the major issues in the area of exercise prescription today is whether an exercise electrocardiogram should be mandatory prior to prescribing an exercise program for an otherwise healthy person. Several years ago, there was a large segment of the medical community that felt that an exercise test was necessary, and it was then the recommendation that an exercise electrocardiogram be included as a part of the medical evaluation of individuals over 35 years of age before beginning an exercise program. While this is a sound and medically justifiable position, it is not very practical. First, most people living in rural communities have little or no access to such a screening test. Even in many larger cities, it is virtually impossible to make an appointment for an exercise electrocardiogram due to the fact that the physician conducting these tests will accept only those with known or suspected coronary artery disease. The time, facilities, equipment, and personnel are simply not sufficient to test all of those individuals who might want to start an exercise program. The second problem relates to the cost of such a test. In most communities, it will cost between $100 and $200 or more for the exercise test alone. This automatically takes the test out of the realm of possibility for those with low incomes. At this point in time, most insurance companies will not pay any part of the costs of this test, unless the person is a referral for suspected coronary artery disease. Lastly, the test yields relatively few individuals who have significant coronary artery disease which had not been previously detected. It is unknown, at this time, how great a risk exercise would impose on these individuals had they been prescribed an exercise program without the benefit of an exercise electrocardiogram. At this time, the best advice appears to be to take the test if it is available and affordable, but to not be overly concerned if it isn't possible to take the test for whatever reason. It would seem that you would be at a substantially higher risk remaining sedentary because of the inability to take an exercise electrocardiogram test than to proceed with an exercise program, starting at a very low level and increasing the intensity and duration of activity at a slow rate of progression.

Contraindications to Exercise

There are certain medical problems which, when present, are direct contraindications to exercise. Under no circumstances are individuals to exercise when they have uncompensated heart failure, a recent heart attack, severe anemia, myocarditis, dissecting aneurysm, uncontrolled diabetes, moderate to severe valvular disease, changing patterns of angina pectoris, and certain arrythmias. There are other medical conditions in which the individual is allowed to exercise, but only under strict medical supervision. Individuals who are likely candidates for medically supervised programs include those who have stable angina pectoris, accelerated hypertension or blood pressures greater than 180 mmHg systolic and/or 100 mm diastolic, cardiomegaly (enlarged heart), arthritis with activity, heart attack after 1 to 6 months, atrial fibrillation when under control, corrected anemia, and those patients who are under specific drug therapy.

Whenever a minor illness, injury, or infection may be aggravated by exercise, the exercise program should be terminated for an appropriate period of time. The presence of a virus always leads to the possibility of myocarditis and sudden death, even in a person with perfectly normal coronary arteries and a high level of fitness. With colds or flu, it is best to stop vigorous exercise altogether until you have fully recovered, particularly when fever is present. Abnormal heart rhythms during exercise should be an absolute warning to stop exercising immediately.

One additional area will be mentioned, but with the realization that the information presented will usually fall on deaf ears: Once a major, or even minor, injury has been sustained, it is important in most instances to slow down or stop activity altogether until the injury has had the appropriate time to heal.

For serious athletes, or even recreational athletes or individuals who are exercising for health-related purposes, one of the most difficult things to do is to slow down or to stop the activity altogether. As was mentioned in the second chapter, exercise can be addictive, and if you deprive individuals of their daily dose of exercise, they actually develop withdrawal-like symptoms. Typically, these individuals refuse to adhere to sound medical advice and end up with a much more serious injury. An injured area must have rest for a sufficient period of time during which healing can take place. Attempting to train through the injury usually greatly prolongs the time necessary to achieve full recovery. If the individual must have some form of activity during the period of convalescence, there are typically substitute activities that can be recommended which allow appropriate activity, but which protect the injured area. As an example, when a distance runner sustains a major knee or ankle injury, it would be foolish and medically unsound to continue with the running program until that time when sufficient healing had taken place. A good substitute activity might be pedaling a stationary bicycle, swimming, or jogging in the pool with the body submerged to the base of the neck. These activities would have to be evaluated very carefully to ensure that they were not aggravating the original injury.

One fear with any injury is the loss of physical conditioning and physiological function during the period of inactivity. Physical deconditioning occurs at a rate which is nearly a mirror image of the rate of conditioning; the benefits are lost at the same rate they were gained. It is therefore imperative for the athletic population to devise methods to maintain or at least minimize the loss of general fitness, including strength, power, muscular endurance, and cardiovascular endurance. A good physical therapist or athletic trainer who is accustomed to working with athletic injuries can usually provide an appropriate plan of action.

Physical Performance Profile

It is quite typical for many of us to go to a family physician for an annual or semi-annual medical evaluation with the expectation that the physician will find something wrong and be able to prescribe some form of medication which will provide an instant cure, unlimited energy, deep quality sleep, and a positive outlook toward life. All too often, we are only disappointed when the doctor tells us that we are in perfectly good health, with no diagnosable disease. We may be a "little overweight" and probably smoke too much, but otherwise we are pronounced healthy. Many of us are disappointed in learning what would normally be considered good news, and some will go to another doctor to seek an additional opinion. The majority of our adult American population falls into this category, where the person realizes he or she is not feeling well, or certainly not as well as is desired, yet the physician is unable to identify any specific disease state or medical abnormality. Dr. Robert Kerlan, a highly respected sports medicine physician in Southern California, has captured the essence of this apparent paradox. According to Dr. Kerlan, the standard medical evaluation is oriented toward the detection of disease, with the patient receiving a final rating which ranges from a "0" to a "−100," "0" indicating the total absence of detectable disease, and a "−100" indicating death. A person with high blood pressure might rate a "−20," a person with controlled diabetes a "−50," and a person who had just suffered a major heart attack as a "−80." Again, the rating of "0" would include the majority of the adult American population. Dr. Kerlan has proposed that is it also possible to rate the individual on an expansion or extension of the medical evaluation scale. The ratings would be extended to include the range from "0" to a "+100," with "0" referring again to the total absence of disease, and "+100" indicating perfect health. This expanded portion of the scale from "0" to "+100" is referred to as the health evaluation, and would include an investigation into the dietary habits of the individual, including sleep patterns, smoking and alcohol intake history, ability to cope with stress and anxiety, emotional and spiritual stability, patterns of physical activity, and a physical performance profile. Several of the components of the health evaluation are also major components of the medical evaluation. In fact, the physical performance profile is the unique feature of this health evaluation, for most good medical histories will provide the appropriate information in each of the other areas.

What is a physical performance profile? This is a relatively new concept, and the present battery of tests is being continuously modified and expanded as new information and ideas become available. Basically, most performance profiles evaluate the individual in the areas of flexibility, strength and muscular endurance, body composition (relative and absolute body fat), and cardiorespiratory endurance. Flexibility tests identify these individuals who have poor flexibility, and are at risk for chronic low back problems or other orthopedic types of

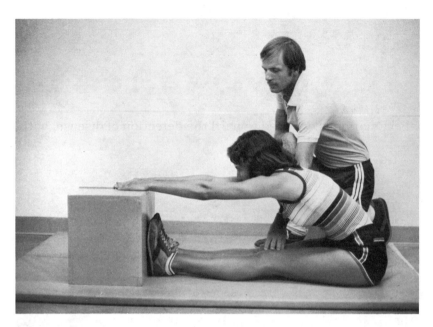

Figure 16 Testing the flexibility of the hamstrings muscle group and the lower back

complications (Figure 16). Strength and muscular endurance can be assessed in any one of a number of ways, using highly sophisticated and elaborate research equipment, or by simply seeing how much weight the individual can lift in a single attempt (strength), which is referred to as the one-repetition maximum; or the number of times the individual can lift a constant weight (endurance). Figure 17 illustrates one of the newer pieces of equipment which is now being used in many research and clinical settings to measure muscular strength, power, and endurance. Body composition is assessed either by the underwater weighing technique or by estimating the body composition from diameters, circumferences, or skinfolds. These techniques were discussed in Chapter 1. Finally, the test of cardiorespiratory endurance provides the most significant information relative to this major health-related component of physical fitness. While each of the other tests is very important and provides useful information relative to the total health profile of the individual, cardiorespiratory endurance

Figure 17   The Cybex II+ strength testing device, which allows an accurate assessment of strength at each point in the full range of joint movement (Photo courtesy of David Hillery, Lumex, Inc., 2100 Smithtown Ave., Ronkonkoma, NY 11779.)

capacity is considered the basic foundation of physical fitness. The best measure of cardiorespiratory endurance capacity is the maximal oxygen uptake, measured while the person walks, jogs, or runs on the treadmill to the point of exhaustion (Figure 18). Maximal oxygen uptake values for average untrained individuals and for highly trained athletes are presented in Table 8.

The person who has stayed in excellent physical condition through a regular exercise program will achieve a very high rating on this physical performance profile. If he or she also had good dietary habits, didn't smoke, consumed alcohol in moderation, got sufficient sleep, effectively coped with stress, and was emotionally and spiritually stable, this individual would rate close to the level of " + 100" on the health evaluation, and would experience the feeling of optimal health and all of its associated benefits. Unfortunately, most people fall far short of optimal health. It is also highly unfortunate that many of these people believe that the way they feel is very

Figure 18 This individual is performing a treadmill test to the point of exhaustion, during which time his electrocardiogram, blood pressure, and oxygen uptake are being monitored.

normal for someone their age, and never attempt to improve their health profile. The health evaluation provides you with objective information relative to where you are presently, and where you could be with a few changes in life-style. Individuals who have been involved in health evaluations are usually amazed when they review their results and find that there is considerable room for improvement. Even more impressive are the positive changes that occur in these individuals once they make the commitment to alter their life-styles and start to see the results of their efforts. It is not unusual to find individuals who at age 50 or 60 years are able to achieve a higher state of fitness and health than that which they had when they were young, and supposedly in the prime of their lives. Figure

Table 8   Maximal Oxygen Uptake Values for Normal Males and Females as Well as Male and Female Athletes ($ml \cdot kg^{-1} \cdot min^{-1}$)

Group	Age	Males	Females
Untrained	10-19	47-56	38-46
	20-29	43-52	33-42
	30-39	39-48	30-38
	40-49	36-44	26-35
	50-59	34-41	24-33
	60-69	31-38	22-30
	70-79	28-35	20-27
Baseball	18-32	48-56	52-57
Basketball	18-30	40-55	43-50
Bicycling	18-26	62-74	47-57
Canoeing	22-28	55-67	48-52
Football	20-36	42-60	—
Gymnastics	18-22	52-58	36-50
Ice hockey	10-30	50-63	—
Jockey	20-40	50-60	—
Orienteering	20-60	47-53	46-60
Racquetball	20-35	55-62	50-60
Rowing	20-35	60-72	58-65
Skiing: Alpine	18-30	57-68	50-55
Cross-country	20-28	65-95	60-75
Ski-jumping	18-24	58-63	—
Soccer	22-28	54-64	—
Speed skating	18-24	56-73	44-55
Swimming	10-25	50-70	40-60
Track and field			
Runners	18-39	60-85	50-75
	40-75	40-60	—
Discus	22-30	42-55	—
Shot put	22-30	40-46	—
Volleyball	18-22	—	40-56
Weight lifting	20-30	38-52	—
Wrestling	20-30	52-65	—

19 demonstrates this phenomenon scientifically. This is referred to as a "bad news-good news" illustration. It is a fact of life that the maximal oxygen uptake decreases with aging, no matter whether one is sedentary, moderately trained, or highly trained. The bad news is that aging is inevitable.

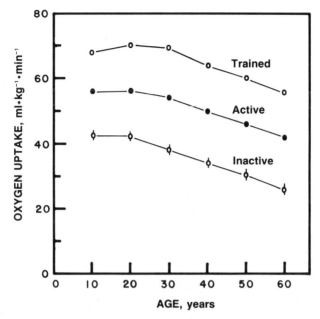

Figure 19 Maximal oxygen uptake in highly trained, active, and in-active individuals with aging

However, the good news is that the person who achieves a moderate state of conditioning at age 50 or 60 years will soon have the physiological capacity of the sedentary 20-year-old. That is truly good news, and may be the eternal fountain of youth which has eluded people for centuries.

4

CHAPTER

Developing a Comprehensive Exercise Program

Over the past decade, the science of exercise prescription has evolved, and has provided a major impetus in getting many previously sedentary individuals back on their feet and into exercise programs which are specifically designed around their likes and dislikes, their abilities and disabilities, their present state of fitness, and to provide them with the optimal dosage so they can achieve the desired benefits. Most people's exercise programs are self-designed; the activity is selected and the person begins exercising. This is a potentially dangerous practice, since most people do not recognize their limitations and are likely to exceed a safe level of exercise. Just as important, people are likely to initiate an activity program without first obtaining the appropriate medical evaluation and clearance. It is highly possible that some people develop symptoms of cardiovascular disease, such as angina pectoris, make a self-diagnosis, and with a fear of their physician confirming their suspicions, they embark on their own exercise program in an attempt to correct the situation. Group programs have associated problems. Although a medical examination may be a prerequisite for participation in these programs, the exercise is typically prescribed on a mass basis and little or no attention is given to individual differences, since everyone is expected to do exactly the same thing. The individualized prescription of exercise avoids these hazards. You receive the appropriate medical clearance, as was discussed in the previous chapter, and your interests and physiologic capacity are individually determined, thus ensuring accurate prescription of an appropriate exercise regimen.

Exercise Prescription

Once you have received medical clearance to participate in an exercise program, you can then be provided with an exercise prescription based on the information from the medical and health evaluations, and the physical performance profile in particular. When prescribing programs of activity, attention must be given to the type or types of exercises or activities recommended, the frequency of participation, the duration of each training session and the duration of the total program, the intensity of effort, and the initial level of fitness. Each of these will be discussed briefly.

Type of Training Activity

A comprehensive exercise program will focus on more than one area of development; thus, most programs include a variety of activities. The foundation of any program, however, must be the cardiorespiratory endurance training activities. This is even true for the athlete who is training for a sport or event which may not involve cardiorespiratory endurance as a major component. Golfers, football players, baseball players, and weightlifters have little need for cardiorespiratory endurance in their specific sport or event, but these athletes as well as athletes in all sports are beginning to discover that a sound cardiorespiratory endurance foundation provides the framework from which they can more effectively develop and execute their skills. For the middle-aged adult who is seeking better health, the need for activities of a cardiorespiratory endurance nature is obvious.

Which activities are appropriate for developing cardiorespiratory endurance? While this will be discussed in substantially more detail in chapter 6, it is appropriate to discuss the major activities at this time. The appropriate activities would be those which maintain the heart rate at its target level for a period of not less than 10 to 15 minutes. Thus, brisk walking, jogging and running, hiking, swimming, bicycling, dancing, and selected individual or dual sports such as handball, racquetball, and tennis, when played vigorously, will all promote improvements in cardiorespiratory endurance capacity. Studies have been conducted which indicate that bicycling and brisk walking provide the same benefits as jogging. Other studies have shown that tennis and racquetball provide improvements, but not to the same extent that you would find with jogging. The fact that the magnitude or extent of improvement wasn't as great with the sport-type activities may not be so important. Improvement was noted, and over a period of years it is quite possible that continued participation in these activities will bring the individual up to an acceptable level of fitness.

Exercise can be divided into two categories: conditioning activities and maintenance activities, although the following concept is awaiting confirmation through research. A conditioning activity is one which is known to provide optimal benefits in a specific area, such as jogging in the area of cardiorespiratory endurance, and weightlifting in the area of strength and muscular endurance. A maintenance activity is one which will maintain the level of improvement achieved through the conditioning activity, and may even contribute to further development of that specific area, but is not considered a primary conditioning activity. In the area of cardiorespiratory endurance, jogging, bicycling, or swimming may be selected as the conditioning activities to increase your capacity from a very low to an above-average level. Tennis, racquetball, or handball may then be selected as enjoyable activities which can be undertaken to maintain, and possibly even continue to improve, your level of fitness.

The concept of differentiating between conditioning and maintenance activities is an attractive one for several reasons. First, it is the feeling of many experts in the exercise and sport sciences that one should get into condition to play a sport, not play a sport to get into condition. While certain sports can be used as conditioning activities, they serve far better as maintenance activities. It is difficult to become proficient in a sport unless you are properly conditioned prior to undertaking the sport. Likewise, it is difficult to improve physical fitness through participation in a sport when you are not proficient in a sport. Second, conditioning activities are very boring to many people. Unfortunately, jogging or running has been consistently used as a form of punishment in the educational setting. Those late to a physical education class, or who were caught doing something they weren't supposed to be doing, were punished by being forced to run a lap or two around the track. It is difficult for most people to reconcile the basic inconsistency between jogging as a form of punishment on the one hand, and jogging as an enjoyable and healthy activity on the other. If jogging were so enjoyable and beneficial, why didn't the rest of the class go out running and make those who were being punished stay back inside the building? Since many individuals simply don't enjoy conditioning activities, and will be early dropouts if they do begin a program which is strictly oriented toward conditioning activities, it has been suggested that conditioning activities be used for only the initial phase of the program. Once you have achieved a pre-set goal for a desirable level of cardiorespiratory endurance, you can then switch to a maintenance activity, which may be more enjoyable and may have a better chance of being pursued throughout your lifetime. Exercise must be a lifetime pursuit. It is not possible for any one of us to exercise vigorously for 2 or 3 years, then live on the residual benefits for the rest of our lives. As discussed in the previous chapter, the physiological and health benefits gained are lost rapidly if the exercise program is discontinued. Therefore, it is important for us to participate in activities that we enjoy and will continue to pursue the rest of our lives.

In addition to cardiorespiratory endurance training activities, stretching exercises can be used to correct an existing problem of poor flexibility, or strength training exercises can bc used to increase basic levels of strength and muscular endurance. These types of activities are appropriate to use in the warm-up or cool-down phase of the cardiorespiratory endurance training program. Simple static stretching and limited-strength training exercises are excellent when used prior to or immediately following the endurance workout, but a major strength training effort should be carried out on a separate day.

Frequency of Participation

With respect to frequency of participation, it would appear that 3 to 4 days per week represent an optimal frequency. In this case, optimal is used to indicate the greatest return relative to the amount of time invested. Obviously, the highly skilled athlete in training for world-class competition needs to be engaged in formal training 6 to 7 days per week. For the middle-aged adult who is participating in the exercise program for its health-related benefits, it would appear that training more than 3 to 4 days per week would provide additional benefits, but the returns diminish once 3 to 4 days per week are exceeded. Several studies have shown that limited benefits may be derived from as little as 2 days per week, but this low frequency is not encouraged.

There is a tendency for individuals who have been sendentary for years, who finally make the decision to start an exercise program, to be overly motivated during the first few weeks of the program. They assume that if 3 to 4 days per week is good for them, then 6 to 7 days a week must be even better. It is far better to restrict frequency to 3 to 4 days per week at least for the first month or two, for the risk of injury or serious orthopedic complications is greatest during this initial start-up period, and the over-enthusiastic beginner may be doing far more harm than good by increasing the frequency. After the first few months of the program when the exercise habit has been firmly established and the potential for injury is reduced, it is safe to increase the frequency to 5 or 6 days per week. If exercise is being used for purposes of weight control, these additional days of exercise will facilitate the loss of body fat.

Duration of the Training Session

It is generally agreed that 20 to 40 minutes per day of endurance training is the optimal amount, again using optimal in the context as defined in the previous section. It must be understood that the 20 to 40 minutes represents the time invested in the cardiorespiratory endurance conditioning activities, and does not include the initial warm-up phase or the final cool-down phase.

Recent theories on the positive addiction of certain physical activities, such as jogging or distance running, suggest that exercise must be carried out for at least 30 to 40 minutes before one receives the "runner's high" and becomes positively addicted to the activity. As yet, this concept has not been scientifically validated, but discussions with those involved in running programs would tend to support these theories.

Relative to the duration of the total training program, you will notice the greatest improvements during the first 6 months of the program. Beyond the initial 6 months, progress will still be seen, but the rate of progress will tend to diminish. Eventually, you will reach the point where there will be little if any further progress unless marked increases are made in either frequency, duration, or in the intensity of effort. There is no reason to progress further once the desired fitness levels have been achieved, so the decision to seek further improvement, or to maintain the present level of fitness, is up to you. Even with the desire to continue to improve, you must realize that you will eventually reach your genetically determined upper level, and that further progress is impossible, even if you were to train 8 hours per day, 7 days per week. It is important to understand this since many people are highly motivated by the improvement they see in the first 6 to 12 months of their exercise program. Many who are on running programs measure their success by how much faster they are able to cover a fixed distance. They become slaves to their stopwatch, and once they reach that point where they can't run any faster, they lose interest in what they are doing and stop exercising altogether. While progress and improvement are important motivators, you must be careful not to depend too much on these factors and must learn to gain intrinsic motivation from the activity itself.

Intensity of Performance

One of the most frequently asked questions by individuals beginning an exercise program is: "How hard do I have to push myself?" This is also the most important question, since exercising at too high an intensity leaves a person totally exhausted and is potentially dangerous for the older individual who has been sedentary for a number of years. On the other hand, exercising at too low an intensity will result in little or no improvement, since there does appear to be a minimal or threshold level of intensity which must be exceeded before improvements can be realized. This minimal or threshold level appears to be somewhere around 45% of the participant's endurance capacity. Most research studies recommend that the intensity be established at between 50% and 80% of the individual's capacity. Past experience has shown that an appropriate exercise intensity is usually overestimated by most individuals, not underestimated. This is typified by the ex-athlete who recalls how hard he had to work as a boy or young man to condition himself for his sport. Unfortunately, this concept carries over into his health-related exercise program. It is, therefore, important to monitor exercise intensity to protect yourself from overdoing it, yet to make sure that the level of exercise is sufficient to result in the desired changes. How can we safely monitor exercise intensity?

Research has verified that heart rate can be effectively used to monitor the intensity of exercise. This led to the use of the term target or *training heart rate* (THR). The THR is an individually determined value that defines the precise heart rate at which you should train. The THR is established most accurately by performing an exercise test on the treadmill or cycle ergometer to the point of exhaustion. This test determines your maximal capacity and maximal heart rate. A THR is then assigned which represents a fixed percentage of that capacity. A THR set at 75% of your maximal heart rate represents a level of only 60% to 65% of your maximal oxygen uptake, which has been found sufficient to produce a substantial training response.

In the absence of a maximal exercise test, it is possible to provide an estimate of the training heart rate by using the following procedure to establish a range:

Training heart rate range
   Upper level: (220 − age) × 0.80
   Lower level: (220 − age) × 0.65

   Example: Age 45 years
   Upper level: (220 − 45) × 0.80 = 175 × 0.80 =
            140 beats per minute
   Lower level: (220 − 45) × 0.65 = 175 × 0.65 =
            114 beats per minute

Since this is strictly an estimate, and may not be appropriate for any one specific individual, it is suggested that you subjectively evaluate how stressful the exercise bout feels starting at the lower level of the THR range. Each day you may increase the intensity by 5 beats/min. if the previous day's exercise session was perceived as being relatively easy. Even when the THR has been precisely defined by a maximal exercise test, it is not unusual for two individuals to perceive this same level of exercise differently. Some can tolerate much higher intensities, approaching 85% to 90% of their capacity without perceiving the exercise as exhaustive or too strenuous, while others have difficulty maintaining the THR which represents only 75% of their individual capacities. It is quite possible that the perception of effort, referred to as the perceived exertion, may well represent a valid training intensity.

An additional technique which has been used to prescribe exercise intensity is that of METS. One MET is the equivalent of the resting metabolic rate. Various activities have been classified according to how many METS are required to perform that activity. As an example, playing singles tennis is considered a 6-MET activity; it requires an average metabolic rate which is six times the resting level. Singles handball is considered a 10-MET activity. The individual's maximal exercise capacity is determined and expressed relative to MET values. As an example, since the resting metabolic rate is assumed to be 3.5 ml of oxygen per kilogram of body weight per minute, a maximal oxygen uptake of 35 ml•kg^{-1}•min^{-1} would be equivalent to a level of 10 METS (35 ÷ 3.5). Taking 75% of the individual's capacity would yield a training level of 7.5 METS (10 METS × 0.75). That individual would then go to that table which expresses all activities according to their MET equivalents and select from those activities which will provide an exercise intensity of 7.5 METS (see Table 19, Chapter 8).

The training heart rate approach for monitoring exercise intensity has distinct advantages over the MET approach. First, several research studies have indicated that the heart rate, by itself, is a very good index of the actual work being performed by the heart. This is very logical since the heart is a muscle, and the faster it beats the more work it has to do, the more energy it needs to supply its demands, and the more blood it needs to supply the increased energy demands. Using the THR approach will assure you that the work of the heart will remain constant irrespective of the conditions in which you exercise. With the MET approach, the total metabolic activity of the body is held constant, while the work of the heart can vary considerably for the same metabolic activity. If an individual had been given a MET prescription of 7.5 METS, this would be the equivalent of jogging at a pace of 5 miles per hour, or 1 mile every 12 minutes. During cool weather at sea level, this 5-mile-per-hour jog would require an acceptable level of work by the heart. However, if the weather suddenly became warm and humid, or the individual flew to Aspen, Colorado, which is at an altitude of approximately 7,000 feet, the metabolic cost of the activity would not change, that is, 7.5 METS, but it would require a considerably greater amount of work for the heart, and, in fact, might exceed the ability of the heart. Exercise intensity should be based on the work of the heart, not on the metabolic level of the whole body. When exposed to these extremes in temperature or altitude, the body simply will do less work to attain the same THR.

One additional advantage of the THR approach over the MET approach relates to the fact that the THR automatically accounts for improvement. One of the classic changes or adaptations associated with an endurance training program is the reduction in heart rate for the same level of work, or, a higher level of work is accomplished in order to attain the same heart rate. With the THR approach, you theoretically have to perform more work or perform at a higher rate of work in order to achieve the same THR. Therefore, THR doesn't have to be adjusted as you become better conditioned. With the MET approach, since the metabolic load is constant, your maximum capacity must be re-evaluated periodically, and the prescribed MET level altered accordingly.

Initial Fitness Level

The initial fitness level of those starting an exercise program is also an important consideration when prescribing exercise. With low endurance fitness you will be started on a much more conservative program. The THR will be maintained at 70% to 75% of your maximal heart rate and the rate of progression will be slow. With high endurance fitness you can start on a program with a THR representing 80% to 85% of your maximal heart rate and you can proceed at a much faster rate of progression.

A Complete Exercise Program

Once the medical clearance has been obtained and the exercise prescription determined, it is necessary to integrate all of the information described above into a total exercise program. The total exercise program should include: a warm-up and stretching period; the endurance conditioning period; the cool-down period; and, if desired, a strength conditioning period.

The warm-up and stretching period is intended to serve two specific purposes. First, it is important to gradually prepare your body for the strenuous endurance conditioning period that follows. Therefore, you should start with low-level activity and progress to more vigorous activity. Improvement of flexibility is a second purpose of this period. Static stretching exercises are integrated with calisthenic-type warm-up exercises to provide 5 to 15 minutes of continuous activity. A sound warm-up and stretching period will help reduce the amount of muscle and joint soreness that is typically experienced during the first few weeks of an exercise program. In addition, studies at the University of California, Los Angeles, have found that individuals who proceed directly into vigorous exercise without prior warm-up will demonstrate serious abnormalities in their electrocardiogram during the first few seconds of this activity. Appropriate warm-up, stretching, and cool-down exercises will be discussed in much greater detail in the next chapter.

The endurance conditioning period is the "heart" of the total exercise program. The exercise prescription, described in the preceding section, outlines all of the details of this period. Once the type of activity has been selected, and the frequency and duration of exercise established, it is important to properly define the THR range. During the initial 2 to 3 weeks of the program, you should stop approximately every 5 minutes in the endurance conditioning period and monitor your pulse rate. The radial artery on the thumb side of the wrist, or the carotid artery in the upper part of the neck, just to the side and slightly above the larynx (voice box), can be palpated with the fingers. Using a wristwatch or clock, count the number of pulses in a 15-second period, and multiply this count by 4 to derive the number of beats per minute. The pulse rate stays elevated at its exercise rate for the initial 10 to 15 seconds of the recovery period, so if the count is taken immediately upon stopping exercise, the derived pulse rate is an accurate index of the true rate during the last few minutes of exercise. If the derived rate upon stopping exercise is below the lower limit of the THR range, then the intensity of exercise should be increased. If it is above the upper limit of the THR range, the intensity should be decreased. After several weeks of monitoring, you will learn to read your body and stay very close to your THR range with only periodic monitoring of the rate.

The cool-down period is extremely important, for the demands of the muscles during exercise have opened up a number of blood vessels in the active muscles. If the exercise was predominantly a lower-body exercise, such as jogging or bicycling, there would be a large volume of blood starting to pool in the veins of the lower extremities immediately upon the cessation of exercise. If you were just to stop exercising and stand in place, this pooling of blood could lead to nausea, dizziness, and fainting. Cool-down exercises combine stretching with active walking, or some other form of rhythmic activity, to assist the blood back to the heart through the squeezing-effect rhythmic muscle contraction has on the veins in the immediate area. This low-level activity also helps to reduce the degree of subsequent muscle soreness.

Special Exercise Programs

There are certain individuals who should exercise only in a structured program under the direct supervision of a physician. The medical problems which would place a person in this category were outlined in the previous chapter. In general, individuals in medically monitored programs follow almost identical guidelines to those discussed above. The major difference would be in the selection of activities, in the intensity of participation, and in the rate of progression. Due to the restrictive nature of a medically supervised program having to be conducted in a relatively small area where all participants must exercise within view of the physician, nurse, or trained technician, this by necessity limits the selection of activities available. Most medically supervised programs provide walk/jog/run activity, swimming or stationary cycling, and equipment for upper body development. The intensity of the exercise is scaled to the nature of the medical problem. If a patient develops significant heart irregularities during exercise at a certain heart rate, then the THR range is adjusted well below this level. Lastly, the rate of progression is very slow for most patient groups. It is far better to be conservative in approach, rather than to place the patient in a high-risk situation. There have been several notable exceptions to this conservative approach. Dr. Terrance Kavanagh of Toronto, Ontario, and Dr. Jack Scaff of Honolulu, Hawaii, both practicing cardiologists, have trained selected post-coronary patients to run in full 26.2-mile marathons. Not all heart attack victims can be trained to this level, nor should they try, but this does point to the degree of recovery some of these patients can attain.

Unfortunately, not every community has a physician-supervised exercise program available to those patients who should be in such programs. What does the patient do? Exercise is considered to be an essential part of the therapy in the rehabilitation of individuals with most of the diseases that are assigned to this category of physician-supervised program. Is the patient safer to remain sedentary and lose the positive benefits of the exercise program, or is it safer to exercise on his or her own recognizing the need to proceed with caution? For most patients, the latter course would be recommended, and, in fact, is the standard approach of most physicians today. If a patient reaches that point in recovery where exercise is considered important, the physician will typically send the patient off on his or her own, starting with very low levels of activity. Obviously, the conservative approach is called for at this point. Exercise should be at a very low intensity and the rate of progression should be very gradual. In addition, the spouse, relative, neighbor, or a close friend should be encouraged to accompany the patient during each exercise session, and should be trained in cardiopulmonary resuscitation procedures in the event of complications. Patients should also be instructed as to how they can closely monitor their body signs and symptoms. When they start to sense that they are having difficulty, they can reduce the intensity or stop the exercise altogether and then consult with their physician to determine if it is safe for them to continue at a later date.

The Educated Consumer

When you finally make the commitment to begin an exercise program, you are suddenly placed in a vulnerable position, at the mercy of those who are trying to sell equipment, books, and memberships in health clubs or fitness centers, just to name a few. The final section of this chapter will deal specifically with a few basic pointers on how to invest wisely.

One of the first decisions that has to be made concerns the location of the facility where the exercise program will be conducted. Obviously, the first, and sometimes best, choice is your home and/or neighborhood. Many joggers take this approach and it works out most satisfactorily for the majority of them. However, if the program includes weight training, or a sport such as racquetball, this may well take the exercise program away from the home and into some community or commercial agency. How do you select from among all of the available choices? It is not unusual to have programs available through the local YMCA, YWCA, YMHA, YWHA, public school, community or state college, university, health spa, fitness center, or sports center. Usually, financial considerations will, by necessity, take precedence in the final decision-making process. However, there are other considerations which need to be resolved as you make your decision.

First, the issue of cost and specifically what is included for the cost must be clarified. Often, costs are hidden, and it is only after the final contract has been signed that the full costs are disclosed. If thcrc are several facilities under consideration, it is wise to conduct a simple cost/benefit ratio. One facility may cost slightly more, but may provide much more in the way of equipment, space, and experienced personnel. Is the equipment available which will be needed in the individualized exercise program? Is instruction or supervision available? Will the facility be open and available at convenient times? Does the facility have an established reputation? Are the instructors and supervisors knowledgeable, and have they been trained properly; for example, do they hold an undergraduate college degree in physical education? These and other questions should be answered before a final decision is made. If there is a state college or university in the local vicinity, there will usually be an exercise physiologist on the faculty who can assist you in making this decision. In many instances, the local state college or university will have established its own adult fitness program. These are typically sound programs with good facilities, well-trained personnel, excellent testing programs, and are usually very reasonably priced.

In 1975, The Association of Physical Fitness Centers was formed by a group of concerned physical fitness oriented companies. The association is dedicated to maintaining standards in health spa, health club, and fitness center operations. They have established a code of ethical practices to which each member must adhere to remain in good standing. The association's national office is located in Suite 500, 5272 River Road, Washington, D.C. 20016, and maintains an active file of its membership. The code of ethics was developed to protect the consumer, so a member organization in good standing represents a sound business operation.

Other decisions relate to clothing, shoes, and special equipment, such as rackets, clubs, and indoor exercise devices. When the exercise prescription specifies games like tennis or racquetball, or an indoor exercise device such as a stationary cycle, proper knowledge of the equipment under consideration is important. It would be impossible in this book to discuss all possible items of equipment likely to be used in an exercise program. However, there are certain guidelines that can be applied in the purchase of most specialized exercise equipment, including the following:

1. Deal with reputable businesses that will stand behind their products.
2. Consult experts in the field, or various consumer reports, if there is any question about a company or its product. Most Ys, colleges, or universities have experts in this area who would be willing to provide assistance.
3. Avoid devices that claim to do all of the work. Active participation is essential to obtain the desired benefits of exercise.
4. Do not be misled into thinking that the more expensive the item, the better job it does. Many items of equipment are greatly overpriced.
5. Do not buy something that will not be used. Many expensive items of exercise equipment end up being stored in the garage, basement, or attic.
6. Do not buy on impulse after receiving a high-powered sales pitch. Wait at least 3 days before making the final decision.
7. Understand completely the purpose of the exercise device and its principle of operation.

Finally, many sports have become so popular that specialized magazines have been started to cater to the specific needs and interests of participants in those sports. These magazines typically provide sound articles and information relative to consumer affairs, in addition to articles on training techniques, strategies, and other areas of interest. As an example, *Runner's World* magazine is a monthly publication for runners of both sexes, all ages, and all abilities. It devotes one issue each year to rating the various running shoes. This is an outstanding consumer service which has forced the shoe manufacturers to improve on shoe design and to produce a better-quality shoe.

In summary, the information is there if the consumers will take the time to ask the appropriate questions and to do a little homework. Literally millions of dollars arc foolishly spent each year because consumers simply did not take the time to become informed. Informed consumers will make reasonable demands on the free-enterprise system, which will only work to improve the quality of products and service over a period of time.

5

The Warm-Up, Stretching, and Cool-Down Periods

The importance of an appropriate warm-up and stretching period and a cool-down period was discussed in detail in the previous chapter. The warm-up and stretching period is designed to stretch the muscles for the purpose of increasing or maintaining proper flexibility of the major joints, and to gradually prepare the whole body for the endurance conditioning period. How important is this warm-up and stretching period? It is not unusual to see athletes bypass the warm-up and stretching period and proceed directly into the endurance conditioning phase. This is also true of many recreational joggers, who simply start jogging without the appropriate warm-up and stretching period. These individuals typically justify their actions by stating that they start slowly, using the intitial part of their endurance conditioning period as the warm-up to a faster pace which follows. What does research conclude with respect to the value of warm-up and stretching?

Most research on warm-up has looked at its importance relative to athletic performance; that is, is warm-up essential in order to achieve the best athletic performance? This question is much more complex than it may appear on the surface, for there are various forms of warm-up. As an example, for the baseball player, there are specific (throwing) and general (calisthenics) activities which are considered active forms of warm-up. In addition, there are also passive forms of warm-up, such as hot showers, massage, or heating pads. With this in mind, the research would tend to indicate that warm-up facilitates speed of movement, range of motion, and strength in movements of selected parts of the body, but it doesn't affect reaction time. Sprints and distance runs are improved with warm-up, but agility runs are not. Baseball-throwing speed and softball distance throw are improved with warm-up, but accuracy of the throw appears to be unaffected by warm-up. Most coaches and athletes feel that warm-up is essential to prevent injuries, but there is very little direct research evidence to support their beliefs. The study referred to in the previous chapter demonstrated significant abnormalities in the exercise electrocardiogram when burst-type activities were performed without prior warm-up. Even though the research literature is equivocal relative to the benefits of warm-up, it would appear wise to include warm-up activities as an important part of the total exercise program until more substantial evidence surfaces to indicate that it could be safely omitted.

Stretching exercises are extremely beneficial in developing increased flexibility. Athletes who don't stretch are much more susceptible to musculoskeletal problems or injuries, such as sprains, strains, and muscle pulls. Certain types of endurance conditioning activities actually work to decrease an individual's flexibility. Most distance runners who ignore stretching exercises are usually able to reach their kneecaps, but not much farther, when asked to touch their toes. Running over a period of months or years will definitely reduce flexibility in the legs and lower back, and will occasionally lead to chronic lower back problems if not corrected.

Flexibility can be increased through rapid or ballistic types of movements, such as bobbing or jerking, or through slow controlled stretching. Using seated hip flexion as an example (see Figure 16), in the ballistic approach you would lean forward at the waist, keeping the knees locked out in full extension, and bounce or bob forward and backward, attempting to touch your toes. In controlled stretching, sometimes referred to as static stretching, you lean forward, grab the ankles, and then very slowly pull forward, placing the muscles on slow stretch. Research has shown both methods to be equally effective, but the controlled stretching technique is advocated since there appears to be less danger of injury and soreness, and the antagonist group of muscles are fully relaxed.

Warm-Up and Stretching Period

The warm-up and stretching period can last from several minutes to 10 or 15 minutes, depending on the need for thorough warm-up and stretching. Those who have acceptable levels of flexibility, and who warm up quickly, may need only a few minutes of stretching and light calisthenics to prepare themselves for the endurance conditioning period. Others may be slow starters, and may need to concentrate on a number of specific stretching exercises to improve their flexibility. Thus, the content of the warm-up and stretching period will be totally dependent on the needs and desires of the individual. The following exercises have been selected as appropriate for inclusion in the warm-up and stretching period. The number of repetitions for each exercise will vary from one exercise to the next, and according to the fitness level and ability of the individual. Therefore, recommendations for repetitions have been established for three different levels: A—beginning; B—intermediate; and C—advanced. You will have to make the decision as to which is the appropriate level for you. Exercises 14 and 15, for example, should be done only after reaching an advanced level of exercise.

1. Head rotation

Purpose: to stretch the muscles of the neck and upper back

Start: standing upright with the hands on the hips, and the feet placed shoulder-width apart

Movement: slowly rotate the head clockwise in a full circle for the specified number of repetitions; then reverse the direction for an equal number of repetitions

Repetitions: A, B, and C—5

2. Head and shoulder curl

Purpose: to stretch the muscles of the neck and upper back, and to promote abdominal strength

Start: lie on the back with the legs fully extended forward, and the hands behind the head or neck

Movement: slowly curl the head and shoulders forward to approximately a 45° position, and hold for 5 seconds

Repetitions: A—4; B—6; C—8

3. Trunk rotation

Purpose: to stretch the muscles of the back, sides, and shoulder girdle

Start: stand upright, hands behind the head, and the feet placed shoulder-width apart

Movement: rotate the trunk as far to the right as possible, and then rotate as far to the left as possible

Repetitions: A—5; B—10; C—15

4. Chest and shoulder stretch

Purpose: to stretch the muscles of the chest and shoulder girdle

Start: stand upright, elbows extended outward at shoulder level, the feet placed shoulder-width apart

Movement: pull the elbows back as far as possible, holding for several seconds and return to the starting position

Repetitions: A—5; B—10; C—15

5. Bar hang

Purpose: to stretch the muscles of the arms, shoulders, back, trunk, and hips

Start: grab the bar with the palms of the hands facing forward

Movement: hang from the bar for 60 seconds

Repetitions: A, B, and C—1

6. Hip rotation

Purpose: to stretch the muscles of the hips and back

Start: stand upright, hands on hips, with the feet placed shoulder-width part

Movement: bending at the waist, rotate the trunk to the right side, forward, left side, and return

Repetitions: A—5; B—10; C—15

7. Push-up, modified and full

Purpose: to strengthen the muscles of the upper arm and shoulder girdle

Start: arms fully extended, shoulder-width apart supporting the upper body weight, with the feet extended backward, the toes supporting the lower body weight

Movement: slowly lower the chest to the floor, keeping the back straight and in line with the buttocks, then push back up to the fully extended position

Repetitions: A—10; B—20; C—30 or more

Note: For those with limited upper body strength, perform this exercise with the knees on the floor forming the point of support. Move to the full push-up when 30 repetitions can be performed.

8. Back hyperextension

Purpose: to stretch the abdominal and chest muscles and to strengthen the lower back

Start: lie on the stomach, with the legs extended to the rear, and the hands behind the head

Movement: with a partner holding the feet, slowly extend the trunk upward as far as possible and hold for 3 to 5 seconds

Repetitions: A—2; B—4; C—6

9. Backward single leg raise

Purpose: to stretch the muscles of the hip and abdomen and to tighten the buttocks

Start: lie on the stomach with the legs extended to the rear, arms to the side

Movement: with a partner holding the hips and lower back in place, lift the right leg up as high as possible, keeping the stomach and hips pressed flat against the floor, and hold for 3 to 5 seconds; repeat with the opposite leg

Repetitions: A—2; B—4; C—6

10. Single knee to chest

Purpose: to stretch muscles in the lower back and buttocks

Start: lie on the back with the legs extended forward

Movement: bring the right knee up and into the chest, pulling the knee with the hands and arms as far forward as possible, hold in the fully stretched position for 5 seconds, and then repeat with the opposite leg

Repetitions: A—3; B—6; C—9

11. Double knee to chest

Purpose: to stretch the hamstrings and lower back muscles

Start: lie on the back with the arms to the side, and the legs extended forward

Movement: bring both knees up toward the head, keeping the arms and upper back pressed firmly against the floor, hold for 5 seconds, and then relax

Repetitions: A—3; B—6; C—9

12. Forward praying

Purpose: to stretch the muscles of the lower back and hips

Start: kneel on the hands and knees, with the knees spread slightly apart and directly under the hips

Movement: keeping the hands and knees in position, lower the buttocks until it touches the heels, and extend the arms forward and lower the chest to the floor and hold for 5 seconds

Repetitions: A-3; B—6; C—9

13. Bent-knee sit-up

Purpose: to strengthen the abdominal and hip flexor muscles

Start: lie on the back with the knees bent to a 90° angle, and the hands clasped behind the head

Movement: curl the head, shoulders and back up to the full sitting position touching one of the knees with the opposite elbow

Repetitions: A—5; B—20; C-30 or more

14. The "Plough"

Purpose: to stretch the muscles of the upper and lower back and hips

Start: lie on the back with the legs extended forward, and the arms extended to the side

Movement: keeping the legs locked into extension at the knees, raise the legs up and over the head, attempting to touch the floor behind the head with the toes

Repetitions: C—3

(This is an advanced stretch)

15.   Kneeling back arch

Purpose: to stretch the abdominal and hip flexor muscles

Start: assume an upright kneeling position with the toes pointed backward

Movement: slowly lean backward, attempting to touch the head to the floor

Repetitions: C—3

(This is an advanced stretch)

16. Pike position

Purpose: to stretch the hamstrings and lower back muscles

Start: assume a sitting position with the legs extended forward and the knees pressed flat on the floor

Movement: grasp behind the knees and slowly pull the trunk down toward the knees, holding the stretched position for 5 seconds

Repetitions: A—4; B—6; C—8

17. Lower leg and heel stretcher

Purpose: to stretch the muscles of the lower leg and the Achilles' tendon

Start: stand upright approximately 3 feet from a wall or post

Movement: keeping the feet flat on the floor, extend the arms forward touching the wall and slowly allow the body to lean forward, holding the stretched position for 5 seconds

Repetitions: A—4; B—6; C—8

18. Groin stretcher

Purpose: to stretch the groin muscles

Start: assume a sitting position, bottoms of the feet together, and the knees pointing outward

Movement: slowly push down on the knees, holding the stretched position for 5 seconds

Repetitions: A—4; B—6; C—8

These 18 exercises represent only a selected few. There are many additional warm-up and stretching exercises which could be substituted for any of the above. Non-cultic Yoga provides an entire series of excellent exercises which help tone and stretch the muscles and tendons of the body. A videotape released in the early 1980s by Raquel Welch, titled "Raquel," is an excellent instructional source for yoga-type stretching. It should be re-emphasized that all stretching movements should be done slowly and carefully. Several of the above exercises are recommended only for the advanced level, since they require extreme coordination and good existing flexibility.

Cool-Down Period

The purpose of the cool-down period is to assist in the return of blood to the heart by simple rhythmic contractions of those muscles used in the endurance conditioning period, and to stretch the active muscles to help relieve existing soreness and prevent future soreness. For the former, it is usually appropriate to continue or modify the endurance conditioning activity, such as walking following a jog or run, or pedaling the bicycle or swimming at a very slow rate. Just as the body is gradually prepared for the endurance conditioning period by a progressive increase in the level of activity during the warm-up and stretching period, it is important that the level of activity be gradually decreased during the cool-down period.

With respect to the stretching exercises to prevent or reduce muscle and joint soreness, specific exercises can be selected from those proposed above for the warm-up and stretching period. All exercises that are selected, however, should follow the initial phase of the cool-down period, in which the conditioning activity or a modification of the conditioning activity is performed at a reduced intensity. Also, these stretching exercises should be performed relatively close to one another in succession, so the body doesn't cool down too quickly, causing you to be chilled.

Assessment of Flexibility

The most accurate tests of flexibility presently available are those tests which assess the actual range of motion of the various joints. However, the equipment necessary for such an assessment is both expensive and not readily available. Also, since flexibility is specific to each joint, no generalized flexibility test is available. However, since most of the medical problems associated with poor flexibility are related to the lower back, a simple test for assessing the flexibility of the lower back is referred to as the sit-and-reach test. This test is illustrated in Figure 16, chapter 3.

In the sit-and-reach test, sit upright with your legs extended directly in front of you, heels spread about 5 inches apart, and knees pressed flat against the floor. A yardstick is taped to the floor between the legs with the 15-inch mark in line with the heels of the feet, the low numbers of the yardstick toward you. Then bend forward slowly at the waist reaching as far forward on the yardstick as possible. The score is taken as the most distant point reached on the yardstick with the fingertips fully extended. The best of three trials is then used as an index of your trunk flexibility and can be compared to the norms in Table 9. It is advisable to have a short warm-up period of stretching exercises prior to performing the test. During the test, the movement should be one of slow stretch not a fast or ballistic-type of movement. Finally, this test is influenced by the length of the arms and legs, but this is not a major problem.

Table 9 Standards for the Sit-and-Reach Flexibility Test

Category	Value, Inches
Excellent	22 or greater
Good	19-21
Average	14-18
Fair	12-13
Poor	11 or less

Cardiorespiratory Endurance Period

Cardiorespiratory endurance should be the major focus of any conditioning program. It is important to recognize that cardiorespiratory endurance is not the same as muscular endurance. Muscular endurance is a local phenomenon, and refers to the ability of the muscle or muscle group to sustain prolonged exercise. The exercise can be either of a rhythmical or repetitive nature, for example, pull-ups or push-ups, or of a static nature, such as in a sustained isometric contraction. The resulting fatigue is confined to the local group of muscles which had been exercised. Cardiorespiratory endurance is a more general, total body phenomenon, and refers to the ability of the total body to sustain prolonged rhythmical exercise. Muscular endurance is highly related to muscular strength, while cardiorespiratory endurance reflects the development and status of the cardiovascular and respiratory systems. Muscular endurance will be discussed in more detail in the following chapter.

Endurance conditioning, which will refer specifically to conditioning to develop one's cardiorespiratory endurance capacity, can be achieved in a number of ways. Probably the most popular form of endurance conditioning at the present time is jogging or long-distance running. There are more than 200 marathon races each year which have been officially sanctioned as 26.2 miles in length, and over 50,000 Americans have successfully completed at least one marathon. Several marathon races consistently attract more than 10,000 starters. But even with jogging or long-distance running there are variations in how one trains. There are those who advocate interval training, where short periods of rest are interspersed with periods of intense work. There are others who advocate LSD training, which is an acronym for long slow-distance training, where the exercise is continuous but at a low intensity. While the following discussion will be largely oriented toward walking, jogging, and running, these techniques are equally effective for other forms of endurance conditioning, such as bicycling or swimming, but they are not necessarily applicable to the various sports which are used as maintenance activities, and which will be discussed in detail in chapter 8.

Training Systems

The major training systems which will be discussed will include interval training, continuous training, which includes LSD training, circuit training, and then a combination approach to training.

Interval Training

The system of interval training, which is presently very popular for training individuals ranging from world-class athletes to patients in medically supervised rehabilitation programs, has had its origins traced back to Germany in the early 1930s. This system was supposedly the result of the collaboration of a coach and a physiologist. Interval training involves the insertion of rest intervals, or, more typically, intervals of reduced activity, referred to as relief intervals, between intervals of work. Basic research in the laboratory has demonstrated that a considerably greater amount of work can be performed per unit time when the work period is broken into short, intense bouts with rest intervals interspersed between consccutive work bouts. The intervals of work and rest are usually equal, and can vary from several seconds to 5 minutes or more. In addition to the terms "work interval" and "rest or relief interval," the vocabulary of interval training also includes the terms "set," "repetitions," "training rate," "training distance," and "frequency." The term "set" describes a series of work and relief intervals. As an example, a typical set might include 8 400-meter runs at a pace of 70 seconds each, with a 60-second period of light jogging as the relief interval. "Repetitions" refer to the number of work intervals within one set. Using the above example, the number of repetitions would be 8. "Training rate" refers to the rate at which the work is to be accomplished during the work interval. In the above example the training rate was 70 seconds to complete each 400-meter run. "Training distance" is the distance of the work interval, or 400 meters in the above example. "Frequency" has the same meaning as has been used in previous chapters, the number of training days per week.

A typical interval training prescription for a single day's workout would be as follows.

Set 1: 6 × 400 meters at 75 seconds (90 seconds jog)
Set 2: 6 × 800 meters at 180 seconds (200 seconds jog-walk)

For Set 1, the athlete would run 6 repetitions of 400 meters each, completing the work interval in 75 seconds, with a relief interval of 90 seconds of jogging. In Set 2, the individual would run 6 repetitions of 800 meters each, completing the work interval in 180 seconds, with a relief interval of 200 seconds of jogging and walking. According to Fox and Mathews in their excellent text entitled *Interval Training: Conditioning for Sports and General Fitness*, the actual stimulus for conditioning is accomplished by manipulating any one or more of the following 5 variables:

1. rate and distance of the work interval;
2. number of repetitions during each set and the number of sets per workout;
3. the duration of the rest or relief interval;
4. type of activity during the relief interval; and
5. the frequency of training per week.

The major advantage of interval training according to its proponents is the fact that you can accomplish the same amount of work and experience less fatigue. As an example, if you were to run as far as possible in 3 minutes on one day, and perform the same intensity of work in 3 1-minute bouts, with a 1-minute rest interval between work bouts, you would have covered the same distance in the same period of time, but the degree of fatigue would be considerably less in the interval workouts. The major reason for the lower level of fatigue is the fact that a different source of immediate energy is being used in interval training which results in the production of substantially lower amounts of lactic acid. Of course, the total workout time will be extended substantially by the addition of the relief or rest intervals. More typically, interval training allows you to do more work in the same period of time; the exercise is performed at a higher intensity.

One of the keys to a successful interval training program is selecting the appropriate intensity or work rate. The THR approach outlined in chapter 4 has been commonly used to monitor work intensity. THR will be established on the basis of the maximal heart rate and the desired intensity. Maximal heart rate is best obtained during a monitored exercise test, or it can be estimated on the track in young, healthy, well-trained individuals. Example:

1. Run one lap around the track (440 yards) at top speed, then monitor the pulse rate during the first 15 seconds of recovery. The 15-second value multiplied by a factor of 4 will provide an estimate of the maximal heart rate in beats per minute.
2. It will then be necessary to determine if the intervals are to be run at 95% of the maximum heart rate (high intensity), at an intensity between 80% and 95% of maximal heart rate (moderate intensity), or at an intensity below 80% (low intensity).
3. In some cases, the duration of the relief interval is dictated by the return of the heart rate during the relief interval to a pre-set level. Once the heart rate reaches this level, the next work interval begins.

For individuals 30 years of age and younger, it is a common practice to allow the pulse rate to drop to a value between 130 and 150 beats per minute before starting the next repetition, and to 120 beats per minute before starting the next set. For those over 30 years of age, since the maximum pulse rate drops by approximately 1 beat per minute per year, it would be appropriate to reduce the above pulse rate guidelines by 1 beat per minute for each year over age 30. The 55-year-old would decrease the above guidelines by 25 beats per minute (55 years − 30 years = 25), and would use between 105 and 125 beats per minute for his or her recovery pulse between repetitions, and 95 beats per minute for his or her recovery pulse between sets. Since absolute accuracy is not critical, it is sometimes easier to take a 6-second pulse count and then multiply the resulting value by a factor of 10. This can result in an error as large as 10 beats per minute, but this is an acceptable accuracy rate for these purposes.

An easier technique can be used to determine the rate of work, and this is largely a trial-and-error technique. If you cannot achieve the desired number of repetitions at the estabished work rate or pace, then the pace is too fast. On the other hand, if the desired number of repetitions is completed and you feel you could comfortably perform additional repetitions, then the pace is too slow. In short, you should be at or near exhaustion by the time you reach the last repetition.

The length of the work interval, both time and distance, will vary depending on the purpose of training. For the elite sprinter, the work intervals are typically short, 200 to 400 meters or less, while the distance runner will concentrate on work intervals that will vary between 400 meters and 1,500 meters or more. Theoretically, this type of training will allow an athlete to complete the racing distance at top speed, without experiencing fatigue or exhaustion toward the end of the run. The number of repetitions and sets will also be largely determined by the sport, activity, or event. Generally, the shorter and more intense the interval, the greater the number of repetitions and sets. Correspondingly, as the training interval is lengthened in both distance and duration, the number of repetitions and sets is reduced. Fox and Mathews have established a series of guidelines which can be followed in the selection of repetitions and sets.

The type of activity during the relief interval can vary from slow walking to rapid walking and jogging, or the equivalent in other activities. Generally, the more intense the work interval, the less intense the relief interval. With increased levels of conditioning, the intensity of the work interval can be increased, or the duration of the rest interval can be decreased.

The above concepts of interval training can be applied to many different sports or activities and should not be considered applicable only to running. In the excellent text of Fox and Mathews, mentioned above, specific programs for various sports are proposed, illustrating how the interval training procedure applies to the conditioning of athletes who participate in these sports. Interval training procedures are also used in the conditioning of previously sedentary adults. However, the work intensity is scaled to their fitness level.

Continuous Training

Continuous training, as its name implies, involves continuous activity without rest intervals. This can vary from high-intensity activity of moderate duration to low-intensity activity of an extended duration. Long slow-distance (LSD) training is a classic example of the latter. High-intensity exercise is typically defined as working at intensities that represent 85% to 95% of the individual's maximal heart rate. For the distance runner, this represents a pace which is slightly below a racing pace; however, this will vary considerably depending on the distance of both the competition run and the training run. There is one major advantage of this type of training. The runner is training at a pace which closely approximates the race pace, and this helps not only in conditioning the athlete, but in helping regulate pace, since running at an even pace has been proven to be the most efficient way to race and should result in the best time. Too much high-intensity training, however, should be avoided since it is extremely stressful and may lead to serious injury. Low-intensity training should be substituted periodically, once or twice per week, to provide relief from this exhaustive form of training.

Low-intensity continuous training is probably the most popular form of training for those who are participating in an exercise program for its health-related benefits. It is popular because it is much less stressful than either interval training or high-intensity continuous training. LSD training became popular toward the end of the 1960s, and its origins have been traced back to Dr. Ernst VanAaken, a German physician and coach who started his initial work on LSD training back in the 1920s. The intensity for LSD training will typically vary between 60% and 80% of the maximal heart rate. Distance, not speed, becomes the major objective. Highly conditioned competitive distance runners who use LSD techniques will run 10 to 30 miles per day, or between 100 and 200 miles per week. Elite runners capable of sustaining a 5-minute-per-mile pace in marathons will train at a 6-to-7-minutes-per-mile pace. There is one major problem with this form of training. While the acute stress is low, due to the low intensity of the workout, the chronic stresses are considerable, and injuries are not at all uncommon. The possibility of injury is a serious consideration for those who are training over 10 miles per day.

Those running under 5 miles per day are not nearly as vulnerable to the "overuse" types of injuries.

The low-intensity continuous training is ideal for the individual who is just starting an exercise program for its health-related benefits. The intensity of exercise is low and is of much less risk than either the high-intensity continuous or the interval training procedures. This is an important consideration since vigorous or burst-type activity in the older individual who has been sedentary is potentially dangerous. The low-intensity exercise is also more tolerable for those who are older or who have not been exercising on a regular basis. The higher-intensity exercises are very stressful and may discourage someone who is attempting to regain regular exercise habits. Low-intensity exercise is typically only moderate to brisk walking for the average 50-year-old male who has been sedentary for over half of his life. It may take him 6 months to a year to advance from a walking to a jogging program using the low-intensity continuous training approach. However, the low intensity and gradual progression may be a major factor in whether that individual adheres to his program or becomes another fitness program dropout.

Another form of continuous training which is used almost exclusively in the training of athletes is Fartlek training, or speed play. Originally developed in Sweden, Fartlek training involves varying the pace from a very slow and leisurely jog to a high-speed, all-out run, but the speed changes come at the will of the athlete. This is a free form of training where distance and time have no relevance. The main goals are fun and enjoyment. This type of training is usually performed in the country where there are a variety of hills, and is most often used as relief from other more structured forms of training. While it is considered as a form of continuous training, the variations in pace are similar to interval training.

Circuit Training

In 1953, Professors R.E. Morgan and G.T. Adamson of the University of Leeds, in England, introduced a new training procedure which was quite popular during the late 1950s and the early 1960s, called *circuit training*. This was an intriguing development, since it incorporated strength and muscular endurance, flexibility, and cardiorespiratory endurance activities into a single program of exercise. Also, it provided a degree of versatility which allowed the program to be varied to meet the specific needs of the individual, or of any one group, such as a group of athletes. With so many positive attributes, it is surprising that this form of training hasn't become more popular. During the past few years, a form of circuit training adapted to the outdoors has been developed and is now being promoted widely throughout the United States. Parcourse is the trade name in the United States, but the concept or idea was originally developed in Switzerland. The Parcourse Fitness Circuit consists of a series of 18 exercise stations, situated varying distances from one another (see Figure 20). From the start of the course, you run, jog, or walk to the first station, where you perform a particular exercise,

Figure 20 Parcourse station (Photo courtesy of F. Richard Cunningham, PARCOURSE LTD., P.O. Box 99589, San Francisco, California 94109)

for example, touching the toes 6 consecutive times, and then move as quickly as possible to the second station, to perform the next exercise, for example, 25 sit-ups. This continues until you have been through all 18 stations. The course is designed to start out slow (warm-up) and gradually build to a fairly strenuous level of exercise (endurance conditioning). It concludes by gradually reducing the intensity of exercise back to low levels (cool-down).

Originally, circuit training was set up inside gymnasiums, exercise rooms, and hallways, or outside on courts, fields, and rooftops. There are usually 6 to 10 stations in a circuit, although this number will vary in direct proportion to the availability of space. The main goal is to complete the circuit as rapidly as possible, with improvement being demonstrated either by a decrease in the total time it takes to complete the circuit, or by increasing the amount of work accomplished at each station, or both. Since the goal is to complete the circuit as quickly as possible, the farther the distance between the stations, the greater the cardiorespiratory endurance conditioning benefits. An example of a circuit training circuit is provided in Table 10.

Table 10   Example of a Circuit Training Circuit

Station	Exercise	Weight, Lbs.	Red Circuit[1] Repetitions			Weight, Lbs.	Blue Circuit[2] Repetitions		
1	Toe touches	—	8	10	12	—	15	17	19
2	Chins	—	1	3	5	—	7	9	10
3	Bench press	60	8	10	12	80	8	10	12
4	Stair climb	—	4	6	8	—	10	12	14
5	Curl	35	8	10	12	45	8	10	12
6	Half squat	80	9	12	15	95	12	14	16
7	Sit-up	—	10	14	18	—	20	25	30
8	Stair climb	—	4	6	8	—	10	12	14

[1]Target time Red-23 minutes
[2]Target time Blue-25 minutes

Various levels are established, depending on the skill level and the ability of the group. In Table 10, the red and the blue circuits indicate two levels, with three steps at each level. The number of levels, steps per level, the range of difficulty for each exercise station, and the specific exercise for each station are determined on the basis of the needs of that group of individuals for which the circuit is being developed. There would obviously be a considerable difference between the needs of a group of high school football players and a group of middle-aged women just beginning a fitness program. In the example provided in Table 10, the middle-aged woman just beginning a circuit training program would start with Red-1. She would complete the circuit three times without stopping, attempting to finish in less than 23 minutes, the target time for the Red level. When she can complete three circuits in less than 23 minutes, she moves to the next step, Red-2. After months of training she will have worked her way up to the Blue level or higher.

Circuit training offers a unique training experience. First, it emphasizes more than one component of fitness, so it could be classified as a total fitness activity. Second, it provides an interesting training environment since there is the opportunity for daily competition against the established times in addition to seeing continuous progress. This would be a challenge and a strong motivation for most athletes. Lastly, the circuit training program can be modified to meet the needs of the individual or the group, and it can accommodate large groups of individuals at a relatively low expense.

While circuit training is traditionally conducted indoors within a relatively small area, the Vita Parcourse idea, which originated in Switzerland, takes the circuit training concept outside. In Switzerland and the Scandinavian countries, the total circuit may be 1 to 5 miles in length, with stations every 400 yards to 1 mile. These courses are typically located in beautiful parks or in the country where there are many trees and hills. The individual walks, jogs, or runs the distance between stations, stops at each station to perform the specified number of repetitions of a single exercise, which emphasizes either strength, flexibility or muscular endurance, and then moves on to the next station.

Combination Programs

Most training programs do not rely exclusively on any one method or system of training, but represent a combination or blend of two or more systems. Combination programs provide variety, and since boredom is a real hazard of any intense training program, this variety reduces the chances of boredom and enhances the chances that the individual will adhere to a training program. For the recreational athlete, who doesn't have the motivation of competition, variety is a very important factor. For the athlete, variety may, in fact, be essential for success. A survey conducted by *Runner's World* magazine, in which the top 20 to 30 runners in each event were polled, indicates that top-level or elite runners at all distances, from the sprint to the marathon, rely considerably on variation. The results of this survey are presented in Table 11. In addition to clearly illustrating the variety in training patterns for any one race, this table also illustrates how differently the athletes train for sprint, middle distance, and long distance events, both relative to types of running and training site.

Table 12 provides an illustration of a combination interval training and low-intensity continuous training program which was designed specifically for individuals who are beginning a walk/jog/run fitness program for its health-related benefits. It starts at a very low level of activity, walking three-fourths of a mile in 22½ minutes, and gradually builds up to a level where the individual is able to run 5 miles in 35 minutes. The rate of progression from one step to the next within any one level will vary considerably from individual to individual. Once the individual has properly identified the appropriate level and step for starting this program, he or she should be able to move from one step to the next every 2 to 4 weeks, if following the program precisely, and working out 3 to 4 days per week.

Table 11 *Runner's World* Survey[1] of the Training Patterns of Top-Level Runners

Race	Ave. Time hr/min/sec	Days/ Week	Miles/ Day	Types of Running[2] (% of each)					Training Site (% of each)		
				S.D.	F.D.	INT.	FLK.	Race	Track	Road	C-Country
100 yards	9.8	5.8	4.8	17	16	49	12	6	50	30	20
220 yards	21.9	5.9	5.0	35	12	39	10	4	37	37	26
440 yards	48.8	5.9	7.5	40	12	35	9	4	44	33	23
880 yards	1:52	6.4	9.0	55	17	17	7	4	28	50	22
1 mile	4:10	6.8	10.5	55	19	15	6	6	22	52	26
2 miles	9:00	6.8	11.0	58	18	11	7	6	17	60	23
3 miles	13:50	6.8	12.8	53	26	9	8	4	18	50	32
6 miles	29:00	6.9	13.0	59	21	10	4	6	18	63	19
9-15 miles	—	6.9	13.0	51	21	5	15	8	17	54	29
Marathon	2:26:00	6.9	13.1	51	25	5	13	6	13	63	24

[1]From World Publications (Ed.). (1974). *The complete runner* (p. 306). Mountain View, California: Author.
[2]S.D. = slow distance; F.D. = fast distance; INT. = intervals; FLK. = Fartlek.

Table 12 A Progressive Walk/Jog/Run Program

Level	Step	Workout Description	Laps[1]	Total Time, Minutes	Total Distance, Miles
WALKING					
I	A	Walk ¾ miles in 22 minutes, 30 seconds	3	22½	¾
	B	Walk 1 mile in 30 minutes	4	30	1
	C	Walk 1¼ miles in 30 minutes	5	30	1¼
	D	Walk 1½ miles in 30 minutes	6	30	1½
	E	Walk 1¾ miles in 30 minutes	7	30	1¾
	F	Walk 2 miles in 30 minutes	8	30	2
WALKING-JOGGING					
II	A	Walk 2¼ miles in 30 minutes	9	30	2¼
	B	Walk ¼ mile in 3 minutes, 45 seconds	1		
		Jog ¼ mile in 3 minutes	1		
		Alternate walk/jog for 5 sets	10	33¾	2½
	C	Walk ½ mile in 7 minutes, 30 seconds	2		
		Jog ½ mile in 6 minutes	2		
		Alternate walk/jog for 2 sets, then	8		
		Walk ½ mile in 7 minutes, 30 seconds	2	34½	2½

	Activity			
D	Walk ¼ mile in 3 minutes, 45 seconds	1		
	Jog ¾ mile in 9 minutes	3		
	Walk ½ mile in 7 minutes, 30 seconds	2		
	Jog ¾ mile in 9 minutes	3		
	Walk ¼ mile in 3 minutes, 45 seconds	1	33	2½
E	Jog 1 mile in 12 minutes	4		
	Walk ¼ mile in 3 minutes, 45 seconds	1		
	Repeat for 2 sets	10	31½	2½
F	Walk ¼ mile in 3 minutes, 45 seconds	1		
	Jog 1 mile in 11 minutes	4		
	Repeat for 2 sets	10		
	Walk ¼ mile in 3 minutes, 45 seconds	1	33¼	2¾
JOGGING				
III				
A	Jog 1 mile in 11 minutes	4		
	Jog ½ mile in 6 minutes	2		
	Repeat for 2 sets	12	34	3
B	Jog 3 miles in 33 minutes	12	33	3
C	Jog 1 mile in 10 minutes	4		
	Jog 1 mile in 11 minutes	4		
	Jog 1 mile in 10 minutes	4		
D	Jog 3 miles in 30 minutes	12	31	3
E	Jog 1 mile in 9 minutes, 15 seconds	4	30	3
	Jog 1 mile in 10 minutes	4		
	Jog 1 mile in 9 minutes, 15 seconds	4	28½	3
F	Jog 3 miles in 27 minutes, 45 seconds	12	27¾	3

(Cont.)

Table 12 (Cont.)

Level	Step	Workout Description	Laps[1]	Total Time, Minutes	Total Distance, Miles
JOGGING-RUNNING					
IV	A	Jog 3¼ miles in 30 minutes	13	30	3¼
	B	Jog 3½ miles in 31 minutes, 30 seconds	14	31½	3½
	C	Jog 3½ miles in 29 minutes, 45 seconds	14	29¾	3½
	D	Jog-run 3½ miles in 28 minutes	14	28	3½
	E	Jog-run 3¾ miles in 30 minutes	15	30	3¾
	F	Jog-run 4 miles in 32 minutes	16	32	4
RUNNING					
V	A	Run 4 miles in 30 minutes	16	30	4
	B	Run 4¼ miles in 32 minutes	17	32	4¼
	C	Run 4½ miles in 33 minutes, 45 seconds	18	33¾	4½
	D	Run 4½ miles in 31 minutes, 30 seconds	18	31½	4½
	E	Run 4¾ miles in 33 minutes, 15 seconds	19	33¼	4¾
	F	Run 5 miles in 35 minutes	20	35	5

[1]Number of laps on a quarter-mile or 440-yard track

Starting such a program involves considerable trial and error initially. First, define your THR or THR range (see chapter 4). Then select the level and step which you feel confident you can accomplish and maintain the THR or THR range. During the first workout, your heart response to this level and step will determine the accuracy of your choice. If you completed the workout with little or no effort, and did not reach your THR, then move up one or two steps and re-evaluate the situation after the next workout at the higher intensity.

Just the opposite approach would be used if you had selected an initial level and step which was above your capacity. Eventually, usually within several workout sessions, you will arrive at the appropriate level and step. Progression from one step to the next within the same level, or from the highest step in one level to the lowest step in the next highest level, is also determined largely by the heart rate response to exercise. As you become better conditioned, the heart rate response to a specific level and step of work will decrease with each workout, although this may not be true on certain days because of complicating factors such as illness, lack of sleep, or increases in the temperature of the exercise environment. Once the heart rate response to a given level and step of work drops 10 beats or more below the THR, it is then time to move up to the next step. It is important, however, not to get overly concerned with time and distance, particularly if they detract from the enjoyment of the activity. For those who work best in a regimented and highly structured program, the program outlined in Table 12 will provide a gradual increase in fitness with many opportunities to monitor progress along the way. Lastly, it is not necessary to progress all the way through this program. Most experts would agree that the individual who is able to achieve Level IV, Step A, has a desirable level of cardiorespiratory endurance fitness. Any progress beyond this point would be solely for the enjoyment of the individual. Some may wish to progress beyond the highest level outlined in Table 12. For these individuals, additional training tips will be covered in chapter 8.

Assessment of Cardiorespiratory Endurance

As was discussed earlier, the best estimate of cardio-respiratory endurance capacity is the maximal oxygen uptake value. This is typically obtained during a test to exhaustion on a treadmill or a cycle ergometer. For the individual 35 years of age and older, this test should be done only under the supervision of a physician. Few facilities are available where one could go to have maximal oxygen uptake measured. Consequently, the only alternative for most people is an indirect estimate of maximal oxygen uptake. Over the past 10 years, research has indicated that the time to complete an endurance run of 1.5 miles or greater has a very close relationship to one's maximal oxygen uptake. Table 13 provides the estimated maximal oxygen uptake for the specific time to complete 1.5 miles. The test can be run on either a 440 yd track (6 laps), or on a 1.5 mile non-repeating course which assures that the total distance was completed, and was not a lap or two short. This test should be given only to those who are in good condition, or who have been conditioned to run that distance. The test is potentially dangerous for the sedentary individual who has been out of training for years. Pre-training is essential for valid results since proper pacing is important for obtaining good results. Those over 25 to 30 years of age should receive the appropriate medical clearance, as outlined in chapter 3, prior to undertaking this test.

Other tests of submaximal intensity have been proposed as valid measures of cardiorespiratory fitness capacity, but each of these has major limitations. A number of step tests have been designed which estimate the fitness level of the individual on the basis of the heart rate response to a fixed rate of work. Unfortunately, these tests have not been found to be accurate in their predictions, although they are theoretically sound. For a given rate of work, the heart rate response of the highly conditioned individual should differ from that of the poorly conditioned, or even average conditioned individual;

Table 13 Maximal Oxygen Uptake Estimated From 1.5-Mile Run Time[1]

1.5-Mile Run Time Minutes:Seconds	Estimated Maximal Oxygen Uptake $(ml \cdot kg^{-1} \cdot min^{-1})$
7:30 and below	75
7:31- 8:00	72
8:01- 8:30	67
8:31- 9:00	62
9:01- 9:30	58
9:31-10:00	55
10:01-10:30	52
10:31-11:00	49
11:01-11:30	46
11:31-12:00	44
12:01-12:30	41
12:31-13:00	39
13:01-13:30	37
13:31-14:00	36
14:01-14:30	34
14:31-15:00	33
15:01-15:30	31
15:31-16:00	30
16:01-16:30	28
16:31-17:00	27
17:01-17:30	26
17:31-18:00	25

[1]Adapted from Cooper, K.H. (1968). A means of assessing maximal oxygen intake. *Journal of the American Medical Association,* **203**, 201-204.

it should reach a lower level during exercise, and it should recover at a much faster rate. Unfortunately, for some unexplainable reason, those step tests which are presently available do not accurately sense the differences in fitness between individuals. Submaximal tests have also been developed for the cycle ergometer. The individual rides the stationary ergometer at two or three different work loads, and the steady-state heart rate for each work load is recorded and is then plotted on a graph relative to the work load from which the heart rate was obtained. The slope of the resulting curve provides an estimate of the relative fitness of the individual, with the steep slope representing low fitness, and the gradual slope representing high fitness. Again, the theoretical basis for such tests are sound, but the tests themselves do not provide very realistic estimates in actual practice. There is a real need to develop an inexpensive submaximal test of maximal oxygen uptake, or cardiorespiratory endurance capacity, which could be either self-administered, or administered by a nurse, physician, or physical educator.

Once the maximal oxygen uptake has been estimated, Table 8 in chapter 3 can be consulted to determine the significance of the resulting value. Generally, a value in excess of 50 ml$\cdot$kg$^{-1}\cdot$min^{-1} for men, and 45 ml$\cdot$kg$^{-1}\cdot$min^{-1} for women 20 to 39 years of age is considered to be very good, and possibly a desirable level to set as a goal if one's present fitness level falls below that level. For each decade above 39 years of age, the above target values should be reduced by 10%. As an example, a 55-year-old-woman would have a target value of 36 ml$\cdot$kg$^{-1}\cdot$min^{-1} (45 ml$\cdot$kg$^{-1}\cdot$min^{-1} − 20% of 45 ml$\cdot$kg$^{-1}\cdot$min^{-1} or 45 − 9 = 36 ml$\cdot$kg$^{-1}\cdot$min^{-1}).

7

C H A P T E R

Training for Strength, Power, and Muscular Endurance

For many years, strength was considered to be the cornerstone of physical fitness. Individuals who spent many hours per week lifting weights, increasing their strength, and developing large bulky muscles were considered to be the epitome of health and fitness. It is now thought that the individual with the highly developed cardiovascular and respiratory systems and good muscle tone represents the gold standard for health. This is somewhat ironic since the focus has shifted from the weight lifter to the distance runner, almost exact opposites in body physique. This change in focus in no way lessens the importance of strength as a primary component of physical fitness. Interestingly, it is no longer unusual for the distance runner to be seen in the gym or weight room working on the development of both upper body and lower body strength. Likewise, weight lifters and body builders are now starting to become interested in distance running!

Throughout the earlier chapters of this book, the terms strength, power, and muscular endurance have been used, but they haven't been clearly defined. These three terms are sometimes used interchangeably, but this is incorrect since each has a distinct meaning of its own. *Muscular strength* traditionally refers to the ability of the muscle or group of muscles to exert force. In most cases, the term "strength" is used in reference to one's ultimate ability or maximum strength for a particular movement. One simple way of quantifying strength is to determine the maximum weight you can lift for a particular exercise, for example, the bench press. Thus, to determine your bench-press strength, estimate a weight you could lift just once, and then attempt to lift that weight. If you were unsuccessful, weight would be taken off until that point is reached when you could lift the weight just a single time. If you were successful the first time, and, in fact, felt you could have lifted considerably more, then weight is added until you reach that point where you can lift that weight only once. This is referred to as the one-repetition maximum, or 1-RM. Assuming two individuals were given the same bench-press strength test, and one had a maximum ability of 200 pounds, while the other attained only 100 pounds, then the first individual would be twice as strong as the second.

Power is simply the product of strength and speed. If both individuals in the preceding example had identical 1-RM bench-press values of 200 pounds, but the one individual was able to push the 200 pounds up to full extension in only half the time of the other individual, then that person would have twice the power for that specific lift, if the distance the weight was lifted was the same. For example, 200 pounds per 1 second and 200 pounds per 2 seconds, over a distance of 2 feet, provides an estimated power output of 400 foot-pounds/second ($200 \times 2/1$) and 200 foot-pounds/second ($200 \times 2/2$), respectively. It is not at all unusual to watch two professional football players square off in friendly competition to determine who has the greatest bench-press strength. Once that contest has been decided, and a clear winner is established, these two individuals will go out to the practice football field, and the weaker man of the two is consistently able to beat his stronger counterpart in line play. Football is a power game, and strength does the player little good unless it can be applied explosively over a very short period of time. Most sports

Table 14 Strength, Power, and Muscular Endurance Compared Across Three Subjects Performing the Bench Press

Term	Subject A	Subject B	Subject C
Strength	100 pounds	200 pounds	200 pounds
Power	100 pounds lifted 2 feet/0.5 second, or 400 ft.-lbs./second	200 pounds lifted 2 feet/2 seconds, or 200 ft.-lbs./second	200 pounds lifted 2 feet/second, or 400 ft.-lbs./second
Muscular endurance	10 reps. with 75 lbs.	10 reps. with 150 lbs.	5 reps. with 150 lbs.

are power sports, and while strength is the primary ingredient of power, the concept of speed must also receive attention. This will be a major point of discussion later in this chapter in the section on specificity of training.

Muscular endurance was defined in the previous chapter to distinguish it from cardiorespiratory endurance. The former is a local factor, while the latter refers to total body endurance. Using again the example of the bench press, where two individuals had identical 1-RM values of 200 pounds, when given 75% of their 1-RM, or 150 pounds, and asked to lift the 150-pound weight as many times as possible, the resulting number of complete repetitions would be a good index of muscular endurance. If one individual could complete 10 repetitions and the other only 5, then the former would have twice the muscular endurance for that specific lift. Table 14 provides a summary of the three terms. While Subject A is the weakest of the three subjects, his power exceeds that of Subject B and is equal to that of Subject C, and his relative muscular endurance exceeds that of Subject C and is equal to that of Subject B. Absolute muscular endurance, which includes the weight lifted as well as the number of repetitions, would be much higher in Subject B, but would be identical in Subjects A and C.

Muscle Training Procedures

Before discussing the various procedures, systems, or specific pieces of equipment that are used to train muscle for improving strength, power, and muscular endurance, it is first necessary to define some additional terms. Essentially there are two major forms of muscle contraction: *static*, or *isometric* contraction; and *dynamic* contraction. Within each of these categories, there are *concentric* contractions, and *eccentric* contractions.

Static muscle contraction, which is more popularly referred to as *isometric* contraction, is that form of contraction where there is no visible movement at the joint, even though the muscles are obviously in a state of contraction. As an example, if you were to walk over to a 500-pound barbell and attempt to lift it overhead, and your maximum strength for that lift was only 150 pounds, you would experience total failure. Obviously, the weight wouldn't budge. You may have applied the maximum force your muscles were capable of generating in that particular situation, but no visible movement of the weight or of the joints occurred. This would be an isometric contraction.

Dynamic muscle contraction is that type of contraction where the joint or joints and the resistance actually move. The lifting of the barbell in the above illustrations of bench-press strength, power, and muscular endurance represent dynamic contraction.

Concentric contraction refers to the shortening contraction of the muscle, while *eccentric* contraction refers to the controlled lengthening of the muscle. This can be illustrated using the example of the biceps curl. The barbell is picked up and brought to rest against the thighs with the elbows locked out in full extension. The curl is executed by contracting the prime flexors of the elbow joint to raise the weight to chest level through complete flexion at the elbow joint. The biceps brachii is the major muscle involved and it performs a concentric (shortening) contraction to raise the barbell to the point of full flexion. The same muscle is responsible for lowering that weight through eccentric (lengthening) contraction. Had the biceps failed to control the return of that weight to the original starting position of full extension, the weight would have dropped rapidly as a result of the force of gravity, and probably crashed to the floor.

In *isometric* contraction, again using the elbow flexion movement as an example, attempting to hold a heavy weight in the palm of the hand with the elbow flexed to an angle of 90° would illustrate an eccentric isometric contraction, providing the weight wasn't too heavy, since the effort was directed toward trying to match the downward pull or force of the weight. With the elbow in the same position, attempting to flex the elbow from the position of 90° flexion to full flexion with the resistance consisting of an immovable object such as a table which is bolted to the floor, would constitute a concentric isometric contraction, providing the table didn't move from its mountings.

When training the muscle, there are various systems or procedures which utilize either static or dynamic contractions. Each of these will be discussed in detail in the following section, but the definition of several new terms or concepts will be attempted at this time. Traditionally, strength training through the use of weights, for example, barbells and dumbbells, has been referred to as isotonic strength training; the term *isotonic* denoting same (iso) tension (tonic). This term is, in reality, a misnomer, since the muscle is exerting different tensions throughout the total range of movement even though the resistance remains constant. However, the term is so firmly entrenched in both the popular as well as the research literature that it will continue to be perpetuated in this book simply for the lack of a better term which has universal acceptance.

Over the past 20 years a new system of dynamic strength training has been developed which uses the term *isokinetic* strength training. In isokinetic exercise, the term loosely denoting same (iso) speed (kinetic), the individual is contracting the muscle or muscle group at a constant speed against a potentially variable resistance. Again, using forearm flexion as an example, the muscles involved in this movement collectively produce a maximal force which is quite different at different points in the total range of motion of the elbow joint. The peak force development occurs at 90° to 100° of flexion. When the muscles contract as forcefully as they can at full extension or full flexion, the force generated is approximately only 70% of the maximal peak force generated at 90° to 100° of full flexion. Therefore, when lifting weights, the heaviest weight you can lift is limited by the weakest point in the full range of motion. Thus, a 1-RM biceps curl of 100 pounds would represent 100% of the capacity of that muscle at full extension, but would represent only 70% or less of the capacity of that muscle at 90° to 100°. In isokinetic exercise, the individual exerts force against a device which is set to move at a constant speed, and no matter how hard one pushes or pulls, or how much force is generated, the device will not move any faster than its pre-set speed. This allows the individual to exert maximal force throughout the full range of motion, providing he or she is motivated to provide maximal effort. Thus, the muscle can exert 100% of its maximum effort at each point in the full range of motion of that muscle, which is one of the basic points of difference between isotonic and isokinetic exercise. In isotonic exercise, the weight which is being lifted is constant, while the degree of effort provided by the muscles, or the relative effort, varies from maximum in the weakest portions of the range of motion, to moderate in the strongest portions of the range of motion. In isokinetic exercise, the muscle always has the potential for providing maximal contraction throughout the full range of motion, and as a result, the resistances will be variable depending on the force exerted by the muscle. This is one of several apparent advantages of isokinetic exercise. The second basic difference between isokinetic and isotonic exercise is the ability to control the speed of movement. In isotonic exercise, the speed is controlled by the relative amount of weight lifted, that is, the closer the weight lifted is to the 1-RM, the slower will be the speed of contraction. With isokinetic exercise, the speed of contraction is pre-set, and no matter how much force is exerted, the speed is maintained constant. This appears to be a major advantage of isokinetic training, but additional research must be conducted to confirm this as fact.

Figures 21 and 22 illustrate two devices which employ the isokinetic principle. The Mini-Gym device (Figure 21) utilizes a rope which, when pulled, is released at a pre-set speed. The speed of rope release is controlled internally and is not influenced by the level of force exerted during the exercise. This basic device can be mounted in any one of a number of different locations, allowing simulation of just about any exercise movement. Figure 22 illustrates a device similar to

Figure 21   Mini-gym isokinetic training device (Photo courtesy of Glen Hensen, Fitness Systems, Inc., P.O. Box 266, Independence, Missouri 64051)

the Mini-Gym, which has been arranged for use on a swim bench. This device allows the swimmer to strength-train out of water, actually working on the patterns of movement used in the various strokes of swimming. This unit has a readout device which provides a direct digital display of the work accomplished with each stroke. In addition, it has a variable setting for controlling the speed of movement. Figure 23 illustrates the Orthotron II isokinetic training device. The Orthotron II unit works on a totally different principle in providing isokinetic exercise. The speed control is accomplished by a hydraulic cylinder which can be altered to allow variation in the rate which hydraulic fluid flows through it; the speed of contraction increasing in direct proportion to the

Figure 22 Biokinetic swim bench (Photo courtesy of Evan Flavell, Isokinetics, P.O. Box 6397, Albany, California 94706)

Figure 23 Orthotron II isokinetic training device (Photo courtesy of David Hillery, Lumex, Inc., 2100 Smithtown Ave., Ronkonkoma, New York 11779)

increase in flow of hydraulic fluid. Finally, the Cybex II + iso-kinetic testing device, which was illustrated in Figure 17 (chapter 3), can also be used for isokinetic training of specific muscle groups.

There are additional training systems which employ dynamic exercise, but which fall outside of the above definitions for both isotonic and isokinetic exercise. These have been classified or termed accommodating or variable resistance devices. Most of these devices vary the resistance by changing the mechanical advantage at various points in the range of motion. Nautilus strength training machines (Figure 24) use an extremely clever technique for altering the resistance

Figure 24 Nautilus variable resistance weight training machine

throughout the range of motion. After studying the maximum force which can be generated at each point in the range of motion for a specific exercise, Nautilus designed a cam which attempts to duplicate the variations in force-producing capabilities of the muscle as it contracts through the range of motion. The cam can be seen in Figure 24. Universal Gym has developed a system for variable resistance training which is illustrated in Figure 25.

Figure 26 illustrates a totally novel and innovative approach to strength training. The CAM II system utilizes pneumatic resistance, which is achieved with compressed air and pneumatic cylinders. This unique approach to training provides a number of interesting possibilities for innovative training procedures.

Finally, Dr. Gideon Ariel, popular exercise scientist in the area of biomechanics, has developed a computerized weight training system. The concept sounds very promising, and

Figure 25 Universal Gym "Centurion," multiple station variable resistance training system (Photo courtesy of Norman Barnes, Universal Gym, Box 1270, Cedar Rapids, Iowa 52406)

Figure 26   The CAM II pneumatic variable resistance training device (Photo courtesy of Randy Keiser, Keiser Sports Health Equipment, 1627 E. Street, Fresno, California 93706)

could lead to major breakthroughs in the area of strength training.

With the above definitions, it will be much easier to discuss specific muscle training procedures. The following discussion will focus on static and dynamic procedures, with isotonic, isokinetic, and accommodating resistance exercises being included under the general category of dynamic procedures.

Static Exercise Procedures

Static training procedures were introduced in the early part of this century, but only gained popularity and support in the 1950s through the research work of two German sport scientists, Drs. Hettinger and Müller. Their initial studies produced some rather remarkable results, indicating substantial gains in strength with only moderate training, with rates of strength increase which exceeded that of isotonic training. When these results first came to the attention of the American public, there was a widespread move to isometric training procedures. In their original work (1953), claims were made that strength could be increased at a rate of 5% of the original strength value per week as a result of one 6-second contraction per day at only 67% of the individual's maximum contraction strength. When contraction strength was increased to 100% of the maximum contraction strength, or when contractions were repeated more than once, there was not a substantial increase in this rate of strength gain.

Subsequent research has been unable to confirm the magnitude of strength gains reported in this original research, but, nevertheless, substantial gains were still observed. These studies, and later studies by Müller and Rohmert (1963), suggest that while one contraction at 67% of maximal strength held for 6 seconds does increase strength, greater improvement will result from 5 to 10 contractions held for 6 seconds each at 100% of maximal strength. It also appears that muscle should be trained in at least 2 or 3 points in the range of motion, since several studies have indicated that strength gains are very specific to the joint angle at which training occurred. As an example, training at a 90° angle in the biceps curl leads to substantial increases in strength at that specific joint angle, but will result in only small increases at 45° and 135°.

Isometric exercises can be performed anywhere with little or no equipment, which is a very attractive feature of this form of strength training. In formal training situations, isometric power racks are very helpful. These racks can be constructed very inexpensively from 4-inch × 4-inch posts which are anchored upright either into the ground or on the floor. Matching holes in both posts are drilled every 6 inches, allowing a steel bar to be inserted through matching holes in each post. The bar can then be raised or lowered to the desired height for any one particular exercise. It is possible to perform almost all traditional strength training exercises with such a rack. The dynamic exercises which will be described and illustrated later in this chapter can easily be adapted to the isometric power rack. Isometric exercises can also be performed in the absence of any formal equipment. Pulling or pushing against immovable objects, and the use of towels, chairs or other similar objects, has provided the necessary resistance to movement necessary to train isometrically.

While the ease and simplicity of isometrics are appealing features, there are also problems which counterbalance some of the advantages. First, because of the simplicity, the individual receives absolutely no feedback relative to the magnitude of improvement. When lifting weights, there is a continuous feedback as to improvement. Bench-pressing 120 pounds, 6 times on Monday and 130 pounds, 6 times on Friday of the same week, provides that individual with specific information on how much he or she has improved during that week. With isometric training, such feedback is not available. This presents two problems. First, it is impossible to determine how much force is being applied at any one time. While the individual may think he or she is performing at maximum, there is no way of ascertaining this. Second, the lack of information with respect to improvement produces a serious problem of motivation. Without any concrete evidence that actual strength gains are occurring, there is the continuous possibility that the individual will abandon this program. Lastly, isometric exercise encourages the use of the Valsalva maneuver, where the glottis is closed and, with a full lung of air, a tremendous increase in intra-thoracic and intra-abdominal pressure is accomplished by contraction of the abdominal muscles and those thoracic muscles involved in forced expiration. The pressure builds to such a level that the major veins, returning blood to the heart from the lower body, either collapse, or their flow is greatly compromised. This reduces the volume of blood returning to the heart, and can result in serious cardiovascular complications. *For middle-aged and older individuals, and particularly for those with suspected or confirmed cardiovascular disease, isometric training should be avoided. The rhythmical contractions of dynamic exercise would be far more appropriate.*

Dynamic Exercise Procedures

Dynamic strength training takes many forms, as was illustrated earlier in this chapter. In general, no matter which system of training, or which specific exercise device is used, there are several basic principles that have universal application. First, the principle of *overload* refers to the fact that in order to achieve a gain in strength, it will be necessary to stress the muscle or muscle group beyond that point to which it is normally stressed. As an illustration, a young boy is hired to load boxes from a railroad freight car onto a truck. The boxes weigh 50 pounds each, and for the first few days they present a real challenge to this young boy. After two weeks of working, he adapts to his job and the boxes no longer constitute a problem. He has adapted to this stress through a substantial gain in strength which was the result of his muscles being challenged by an overload. If the company for which this young boy works suddenly decides to shift to larger and heavier boxes, he will be in another situation where he is overloaded, and he will experience further gains in strength as he accommodates to this new level of work. The muscles must be loaded beyond those levels at which they normally work for significant increases in strength to occur.

The second and related principle of importance when training for gains in strength is the principle of *progressive resistance exercise*. This principle is best illustrated by a story from Greek mythology. According to legend, Milo of Crotona desired to be the strongest man in the world. In his youth, he began lifting a newborn bull once a day, and continued this daily ritual until the bull had achieved full size. Milo eventually became strong enough to lift the full-grown bull onto his shoulders and parade around the arena to the cheers of the crowds. As a muscle, or muscle group, becomes stronger, a proportionally greater resistance is required to continue to stress the muscle to the same degree to achieve further increases in strength. Progressive resistance exercise simply refers to the systematic increase in resistance as the individual increases his or her strength. This principle applies to all forms of strength training and is closely related to the principle of overload.

In 1945, Thomas DeLorme published a paper in a medical journal which was to form the basic foundation for the development of systematic dynamic training procedures. While his initial interests were in physical medicine and rehabilitation, his system of exercise became widely accepted among athletes and others interested in strength training. DeLorme, and later DeLorme and Watkins (1948), proposed a system which emphasized the use of heavy resistance and low repetition, with the intent of increasing strength, power, and the volume of muscle or muscle mass. The initial recommendation was for the individual to perform 70 to 100 repetitions over 7 to 10 sets of 10 repetitions per set. This was later revised to three sets of 10 repetitions each. With this system, it is first necessary to determine the 10 repetition maximum (10-RM), the greatest amount of weight the individual can lift for 10, but no more than 10, consecutive repetitions. The first set is then performed at a resistance of 50% of the 10-RM; the second set at 75% of the 10-RM; and the last set at 100% of the 10-RM. As strength increases, the number of repetitions that can be performed is increased, and when 15 repetitions or more are attained, a new 10-RM is established and the weights used for each set are adjusted accordingly. As an example, if in the bench press, the 10-RM was 100 pounds, then the first set would be performed at 50 pounds, the second set at 75 pounds, and the third set at 100 pounds. If, after 2 weeks, the 10-RM increased to 120 pounds, then the weights for each set would be readjusted to 60 pounds for the first set, 90 pounds for the second, and 120 pounds for the third. Weights are usually adjusted every 1 to 3 weeks, depending on the initial level of strength of the individual, the intensity of training, and the overall potential for further gains in strength. The degree of improvement from one week to the next will vary considerably not only between individuals but also between any two exercises in the same individual.

While the DeLorme technique is still considered to be the basic technique in dynamic strength training, there have been many modifications. The Oxford technique was proposed in 1951 as an alternative to the DeLorme technique. In the Oxford technique, the individual performs 100 repetitions in 10 sets of 10 repetitions each. The first set is performed at 100% of the 10-RM, and each subsequent set is performed at a proportionally lower percentage of the 10-RM, allowing for the development of muscle fatigue. This technnique has also been modified to a fewer number of total repetitions, usually distributed over 3 to 4 sets. In each set, the individual performs the maximum number of repetitions possible, so fatigue is progressive and accumulative.

Based on extensive reviews of the existing literature, it would appear that dynamic exercise should be performed at 5-RM to 7-RM, for 3 sets each training session, 3 to 5 training sessions per week. This will optimize gains in strength and power. To optimize gains in muscular endurance, it will be necessary to increase the number of repetitions per set to 10 or more, and the amount of weight lifted would have to be adjusted accordingly.

As was described in the previous section, dynamic exercise encompasses a rather broad spectrum of training procedures, systems, and devices, from free weights (isotonic), to hydraulic cylinders (isokinetic), to air-resisted movements (variable resistance). The natural question to ask is: Which system and/or device will provide the greatest benefits? At the present time, each system has its own group of loyal adherents which makes many claims for the superiority of one system over another. Are these claims justified? From the limited research which has been conducted to date, no single system of exercise or specific piece of strength training equipment has been proven to be any more effective than any other relative to the ability of the system or the equipment to effect changes in muscular strength. It is entirely possible that the few studies which have been conducted have not asked the appropriate questions, or may not have been optimally designed to answer the appropriate questions. However, until such time that independent research can demonstrate a clear distinction between the results of training on one specific system or piece of equipment compared to one or more of the other systems or pieces of equipment, it must be concluded that no one system or piece of equipment is distinctly superior.

With all systems of dynamic exercise providing essentially the same degree of improvement in strength, how, then, does static exercise compare to dynamic exercise?

- From the limited research that has been conducted, it can be concluded that both static and dynamic strength training produce substantial gains in muscular strength, with little or no difference between the two procedures.
- Static procedures can be used during a period of convalescence from injury, since they, by definition, do not involve joint movement. This will greatly reduce the decrease in size and strength of a muscle or muscle group which typically accompanies inactivity.
- Due to the fact that static procedures will result in strength increases in only a limited portion of the range of motion, dynamic procedures will produce a more uniform gain in strength.
- Finally, dynamic procedures have been proven to be more effective in increasing both muscular endurance and muscular hypertrophy.

The following exercises have been selected to represent a balanced dynamic strength training program to be used with free weights. When other equipment is available, these same exercises can usually be modified to the specific piece of equipment, although the recommendations of the manufacturer of the specific equipment should be carefully followed. When strength training machines are available, they are suggested in preference over free weights for those just beginning strength training, strictly on the basis of safety. Free weights can be very dangerous if the proper precautions are not taken. When using free weights, there should always be at least one spotter, and preferably two, available to hand the weight to the individual when in the correct starting position, to control the weight during the lift, and to take the weight from the individual at the end of the lift. Without spotters, even the experienced lifter can get into trouble as he or she gets tired and loses control of the weight. Most machines either have the weights controlled in a weight stack, or have eliminated weights altogether. The muscles referred to in the description of each exercise are illustrated in appendix A.

Barbell, Dumbbell, and Machine Exercises

1. Standing military press

Purpose: to strengthen the muscles of the shoulder and upper arm: deltoids, pectoralis major, latissimus dorsi, and triceps

Start: stand upright with the feet shoulder-width apart, the weight evenly distributed between both arms and held at chest level with the elbows directly under the bar, using an overhand grip, hands spread shoulder-width apart

Movement: with the back straight, press the weight straight up over the head locking the elbows out at full extension, and return the bar to chest level

Note: isolate the lift to the upper body, keeping the knees locked out in extension and the trunk and back perfectly straight. Specifically, *do not arch the back.*

2. Behind the neck press

Purpose: to strengthen the muscles of the upper arm and shoulder: deltoids, triceps, and upper trapezius

Start: identical to the Standing Military Press

Movement: with the back straight, press the weight up over the head to full extension of the elbows, and return to a position behind the head, touching the base of the neck prior to lifting the weight for the subsequent repetition; following the last repetition, return the weight to the original starting position

Note: adhere to the same precautions noted for the Standing Military Press

3. Bench press or inclined press

Purpose: to strengthen the muscles of the chest and upper arm: deltoids, triceps, pectoralis major, and latissimus dorsi

Start: lie on a narrow bench with the feet spread apart on the floor, the weight held over the chest with the elbows locked in full extension, using an overhand grip, hands spread shoulder-width apart

Movement: carefully lower the weight to the chest, making brief and light contact with the chest, then push upward returning the weight to its original starting position

Note: isolate the movement to the muscles of the shoulders and arms, taking particular caution not to arch the back; the inclined press is performed in the same manner, except the bench is inclined to a 45- to 60-degree angle

5. Bent rowing

4. Upright rowing

Purpose: to strengthen the muscles of the shoulder and arm: trapezius, deltoids, biceps, brachioradialis, and brachialis

Start: stand upright, feet spread shoulder-width apart, and grab the bar with an overhand grip, hands spread approximately 6 to 8 inches apart, bar resting at waist level

Movement: lift the bar to the height of the chin with the elbows directed outward and return to the starting position

Note: isolate the muscles of the shoulder and upper arm; do *not* involve the back

Purpose: to strengthen the muscles of the shoulder girdle and upper arm: trapezius, latissimus dorsi, rhomboids, deltoids, biceps, brachioradialis, and brachialis

Start: bend forward at the waist, back parallel to the ground, knees bent forward to approximately a 45° angle, and grab the bar with an overhand grip, hands spread shoulder-width apart, allowing the bar to hang down; place the forehead on something stationary, for example, a wall, to help remove the involvement of the back

Movement: with the bar hanging at full extension of the elbows, lift the bar upward until it makes brief and light contact with the chest, and return to the starting position

Note: do *not* involve the back

6.   Two-arm curl

Purpose: to strengthen the muscles of the arm: biceps and brachioradialis

Start: stand upright with the feet spread shoulder-width apart, the weight held at the waist or upper thigh level with an underhand grip, hands spread shoulder-width apart

Movement: lift the bar to a position of full flexion and return to a position of full extension

Note: isolate the movement to the arms: *do not* allow the back to arch

7.   Reverse curl

Purpose: to strengthen the muscles of the arm: biceps, brachialis, and brachioradialis

Start: identical to the Two-Arm Curl, except use an overhand grip

Movement: identical to the Two-Arm Curl

Note: identical to the Two-Arm Curl

8. Lat machine pull-down

Purpose: to strengthen the muscles of the shoulder girdle and back: latissimus dorsi, trapezius, and pectoralis major

Start: sit on a bench or kneel on the knees, keeping the back and head upright, grab the bar with an overhand grip, hands spread shoulder-width or farther apart

Movement: pull the bar down to a position where it just touches briefly the base of the neck and then allow the bar to return slowly to its original overhead position

Note: it may be necessary to anchor the feet or legs in some manner if the individual is particularly strong, to keep the weight from pulling the individual up

9. Lat machine triceps extension

Purpose: to strengthen the muscles of the arms: deltoids and triceps

Start: stand upright with the feet spread shoulder-width apart, grab the bar at chest level with an overhand grip, hands close together

Movement: press the bar downward to a position of full elbow extension and allow the bar to return slowly to its original position

10. Bent-arm pull-over

Purpose: to increase the strength of the muscles of the chest: deltoids, pectoralis major, latissimus dorsi, and serratus anterior

Start: lie supine on a narrow bench, with the head at the very edge of the bench, grab the bar with an overhand grip, hands shoulder-width apart, with the arms fully extended overhead

Movement: lower the bar slowly behind the head and downward as far as possible with the elbows coming to a position of full flexion; then return the bar to the original position with the elbows locked overhead in full extension

Note: be extremely careful with this lift, as the weight moves directly over the face

11. Half-squat

Purpose: to strengthen the muscles of the lower back and legs: gluteus maximus, quadriceps femoris, abdominals, and erector spinae

Start: stand erect with the bar resting comfortably on the shoulders using an overhand grip, with the hands and feet spread shoulder-width apart

Movement: lower the weight by bending at the knees to a 90° angle and return to the upright position

Note: padding of the bar may be necessary to keep the bar from digging into the shoulders; do not exceed 90° of flexion. Have full control of the weight.

12. Hack squat

Purpose: same as the Half-Squat

Start: same as the Half-Squat, except the weight is held behind the legs

Movement: same as the Half-Squat

13. Leg extension

Purpose: to strengthen the muscles of the upper leg: quadriceps femoris group

Start: sit on the edge of the leg extension machine with the knee flexed to 90°

Movement: extend the leg outward at the knee joint until it locks into full extension and then return to the starting position

14. Leg flexion

Purpose: to strengthen the muscles of the upper leg: hamstrings and gluteus maximus

Start: lie on the leg flexion machine in the prone position with the knees fully extended backward

Movement: flex the leg at the knee joint to a position of full flexion and then return to the starting position

15. Weighted sit-up

Purpose: to strengthen the muscles of the trunk: rectus abdominus and obliques

Start: lie supine on an inclined board, knees bent to 45°, and a weight held behind the neck

Movement: curl forward and upward slowly, touching the elbows to the knees, and then return to the starting position

16. Lateral arm raises

Purpose: to strengthen the muscles of the shoulder: deltoids, trapezius, and serratus anterior

Start: stand upright, feet shoulder-width apart, dumbbells hanging downward along the side of the body

Movement: raise both arms out to the side of the body to an overhead position, maintaining the elbows locked in full extension, and return to the starting position

17. Bench-lying lateral arm raises

Purpose: to strengthen the shoulders and chest: deltoids, pectoralis major, and serratus anterior

Start: lie supine on a bench with the arms extended outward to the side, and the dumbbells grasped firmly in each hand

Movement: raise the arms sideward to the overhead position, keeping the elbows locked in full extension, and return to the starting position

18. Neck flexion

Purpose: to strengthen the muscles of the neck and shoulders

Start: sit in a chair with the neck in a hyperextended position and the weight attached to a head harness at the rear of the head

Movement: slowly curl the head forward to the upright position and return to the position of hyperextension

Note: control all movement very carefully by making all movements slow and deliberate

19. Neck extension

Purpose: to strengthen the muscles of the neck and shoulders

Start: lie on the edge of a table in the prone position with the head extended out over the edge of the table in a semi-flexed position with the weight attached to a head harness

Movement: slowly pull the head backward into a position of hyperextension and return to the starting position

Note: control all movement very carefully, by making all movements slow and deliberate

Muscle Soreness

There are essentially two types of muscle soreness. Immediately following a bout of intense muscular exercise, there is a transient soreness which may last from a few minutes to a period of several hours. This immediate soreness is probably the result of the accumulation of the waste products of anaerobic metabolism, and tissue edema, or swelling of the local area, due to the high hydrostatic pressures which force fluid out of the blood and into the surrounding tissue. This is the "pumped-up" feeling that the athlete experiences shortly after an intense exercise bout. The pain and soreness in this immediate acute phase is minor and causes little discomfort. Of greater significance is the pain and soreness which is usually felt from 12 to 48 hours following an intense bout of exercise. This pain and soreness can be incapacitating.

The muscle soreness which is felt from 12 to 48 hours after the bout of exercise is now the focus of considerable research. Several early theories were advanced, but they don't appear to be able to account for all forms of this late appearing muscle soreness. One theory states that soreness is the result of small tears in either or both the muscle and connective tissue. While actual structural damage is a possible outcome of certain types of exercise, it is difficult to accept that all exercises where latent muscle soreness has resulted could lead to this level of micro-trauma. A second theory, proposed by Professor Herbert deVries of the University of Southern California (1980), has been referred to as the muscle spasm theory. According to this theory, exercise leads to inadequate blood supply to muscle, which causes immediate pain. This pain generates reflexes for increased motor activity, creating increased local muscle tension, which decreases blood supply even more. He has collected research data in support of this theory, including the finding that static stretching not only helps to prevent muscle soreness, but it also provides relief to soreness when it is present.

Two factors have direct relevance to the eventual discovery of the cause of muscle soreness. First, muscle soreness is usually only present in the initial stages of training, the first week or two, after which it tends to disappear. This observation is valid only if the training stimulus remains constant, for whenever there is a big increase in the training stimulus, there is renewed soreness. Secondly, there appears to be little or no muscle soreness associated with exercises which employ purely concentric contraction. Certain isokinetic equipment employ only concentric contraction, and no matter how hard one trains, there is little or no resulting muscle soreness. In one study, two groups of young men strength-trained isotonically using only the bench-press exercise. One group trained in the conventional way and had the usual amount of muscle soreness during the first few weeks of the study. The second group performed only the concentric phase of the bench-press exercise, lifting the weight up. Two spotters standing on either side of the weight took the weight at the end of the full extension and lowered it back to the individual's chest, thus removing the eccentric phase. This group had essentially no muscle soreness. More recent studies (Armstrong, 1984) have confirmed that eccentric contraction is the major stimulus for muscle soreness, and this type of soreness is associated with microtrauma of the muscle fibers.

Specificity of Training

For most sports or activities, the closer the training activity mimics the sport activity, the greater will be the resulting benefits. Swim training greatly benefits the swimmer, but has little or no positive value for the runner, skier, or cyclist. Likewise, practice shooting of free throws does little or nothing for one's tennis serve, or putting game in golf, but it has big payoffs for the basketball player. How does this theory of specificity relate to strength training, when improved performance, not solely strength development, is the main objective?

The research to date does not support conclusively the concept of specificity in strength training, although the trend is definitely in that direction. If specificity does exist in strength training, what are the implications for designing strength training programs for each sport, or event within a sport? First, the strength training activity should approximate as closely as possible the movement pattern of the sport or event. As an example, the swim bench illustrated in Figure 22 was designed to allow swimmers to strength-train using almost identical stroke patterns that would be used in the water. Secondly, the strength training activity should be performed at a speed which approximates the speed of movement performed in the sport or activity. Since it would be literally impossible to strength-train at the very high speeds of movement that comprise most sport activities, it is then desirable to train at as high a speed as possible. Many of the more recent pieces of equipment have an adjustment which allows variation in the speed of training. For those devices without speed control, the resistance is simply reduced to allow for faster contractions. It is postulated that the high-speed training is essential for the optimal development of power.

Since the theory of specificity is not fully confirmed in the area of strength training, it would appear wise to build a solid foundation of traditional strength development first, and then venture into more specific training. A combination of general and specific training may well provide the best all-around benefits for athletic performance. The ultimate criteria of success from any strength training program which is being used to better prepare an athlete for a sport is the improvement in performance in that sport. To gain strength without an improvement in performance would indicate that the strength training program was an inefficient use of time.

Assessment of Strength, Power, and Muscular Endurance

In the research laboratory, a number of instruments have been devised to assess strength, power, and muscular endurance. The Cybex II+ isokinetic testing device, which is illustrated in Figure 17, is one of the more sophisticated testing devices available, providing a graphic recording of the individual's torque or strength at each point in the range of motion; a curve from which power can be estimated, and a recording of sequential contractions showing the onset of fatigue, which is an index of muscular endurance. Tensiometers and dynamometers are also laboratory devices for assessing peak muscular strength.

One of the best tests of functional strength, however, is the one repetition maximum (1-RM), which was defined in the introduction to this chapter as the greatest amount of weight the individual can lift just once, for any one specific exercise. The procedure for measuring the 1-RM for any one lift or exercise was detailed earlier. Table 15 provides what are considered to be optimal 1-RM strength values for males and females on the basis of body weight, for the bench press, standing press, curl, and leg press. Since strength decreases with age starting at about 40 years, these optimal values should be reduced by 10% for each decade beyond 30 to 39 years: for 40 to 49 reduce values by 10%, 50 to 59 reduce by 20%, 60 to 69 reduce by 30%, and 70 to 79 reduce by 40%.

Power is very difficult, if not impossible, to measure outside the laboratory. Tests such as vertical jump, standing long jump, and softball throw for distance have been referred to as power tests, but their validity as power tests has yet to be established. Consequently, a simple power test cannot be suggested at this time, though current research will provide one in the near future. Muscular endurance can be measured by a number of field tests, including the maximum number of push-ups, pull-ups, and sit-ups performed in a set period of time, for example, 60 seconds. Another technique for measuring muscular endurance, which on the surface appears to be a purer measure of endurance, is to determine how many complete repetitions one can perform prior to fatigue or exhaustion, using a fixed percentage of the individual's 1-RM for that particular lift. This concept was also discussed in the introduction to this chapter. While this appears to be a valid concept, norms do not presently exist since this is a rather new idea. Limited data, however, would suggest that 20 to 25 repetitions would be acceptable when lifting 70% of the 1-RM for any one specific lift.

Table 15 Optimal Strength Values (lbs.) for Various Body Weights (based on the 1-RM test)

Body Weight lbs.	Bench Press		Standing Press		Curl		Leg Press	
	Male	Female	Male	Female	Male	Female	Male	Female
80	80	56	53	37	40	28	160	112
100	100	70	67	47	50	35	200	140
120	120	84	80	56	60	42	240	168
140	140	98	93	65	70	49	280	196
160	160	112	107	75	80	56	320	224
180	180	126	120	84	90	63	360	252
200	200	140	133	93	100	70	400	280
220	220	154	147	103	110	77	440	308
240	240	168	160	112	120	84	480	336

Sport and Recreational Activities

One of the major problems in staying motivated to exercise is that many individuals simply cannot generate sufficient enthusiasm for exercise when their exercise program consists solely of conditioning-type activities such as jogging/running, calisthenics, and strength-training exercises. Conditioning-type activities tend to be boring to many people, and, as a result, the rate of dropout from programs that emphasize such activities is extremely high. Alternative forms of exercise which provide identical or similar benefits need to be identified and promoted. Sport and recreational activities are natural substitutes for conditioning-type activities, since they are pursued with the attitude of having fun. For most people, jogging is work, and as such is boring, while three sets of tennis is play, and is highly enjoyable. For a few people, activities like jogging are considered fun and enjoyable, but these people are presently in the minority. Our society has been recently brainwashed into believing that the only exercises which will truly benefit them are the conditioning-type exercises. Even more specifically, the misconception that any exercise or activity short of jogging is of little or no value has been widely promoted. Those in the majority, who do not like conditioning-type activities, hearing such claims, simply elect to remain sedentary. This is highly unfortunate, for there is a great deal to be gained from sport and recreational activities when pursued vigorously and regularly.

As was discussed in chapter 4, one can either play the sport or recreational activity to get into shape, or get into shape to play the sport or recreational activity. Even though motivation in the early stages of the program may be a significant problem, most experts now agree that it is a far better practice to spend several weeks to several months in basic conditioning activities to establish a desired level of fitness prior to undertaking a specific sport or recreational activity. Skiing, which is one of America's favorite winter sports, is an excellent example. Most skiers, even at the novice level, would not even think about getting out on the slopes without several weeks of pre-conditioning exercises, consisting of exercises to improve flexibility, strength, muscular endurance, and cardiorespiratory endurance. The same should be true for all sport and recreational activities. Attaining a reasonable level of fitness through conditioning-type activities should result in fewer injuries, increased ability to learn the fine points of the sport, game, or activity (basic coordination), and should allow the individual to obtain a greater degree of enjoyment from the activity. Using the sport or recreational activity to get into shape often leads to injury, and can lead to serious, even fatal, medical complications, primarily of cardiovascular origin. A fatal heart attack on the tennis court, or in the racquetball court, might have been prevented had the person achieved a reasonable level of fitness prior to seriously pursuing the sport.

Rating Sports and Recreational Activities

In the fall of 1972, the Opinion Research Corporation of Princeton, New Jersey, conducted a personal interview research survey of the exercising habits of the American population, sponsored by the President's Council on Physical Fitness and Sports. This survey included 1,939 men and 1,936 women, 22 years of age or over and the results were projected to the total United States adult population. On the basis of this survey, some rather striking findings surfaced. First, of those surveyed 45% did not engage in physical activity for the purpose of exercise. These sedentary individuals tended to be older, less well educated, and less affluent than those who did exercise. When asked if they participated in any of a list of conditioning-type activities, the response, by age, is presented in Table 16. These figures are misleading, however, for they do not provide the important information as to how frequently these activities were engaged in, how much time was invested per exercise session, and the intensity at which the exercise was pursued. As an example of the problems associated with such data, of those who said they walked for exercise, which was the most popular form of exercise, over half walked at least one to two times per week, but a substantial number walked less than once per week. For those individuals that participated in sport or recreational activities, bowling was the most popular sport represented by 20% of the total American population, with nearly half of these involved in organized league or tournament play. Swimming ranked second, with 18% of the population as participants, although approximately one-half of these individuals swam less than 1 day per week. Of the remaining popular sports or recreational activities, golf involved 9% of the population; softball, 8.5%; tennis, 6%; volleyball, 5%; water skiing, 3%; and skiing, 2%.

Table 16 Adult Participation in Conditioning-Type Activities for Age Groups by Percentage[1]

Exercise	Age Groups, Years				
	22-29	30-39	40-49	50-59	60 and above
MEN					
Walking	36	27	39	39	46
Bicycling	28	17	18	13	4
Swimming	25	23	15	14	4
Calisthenics	23	13	10	10	5
Jogging	19	8	8	6	2
Weight training	16	6	3	2	1
WOMEN					
Walking	51	45	41	38	33
Bicycling	28	31	20	10	2
Calisthenics	22	17	16	9	6
Swimming	17	16	13	5	4
Jogging	7	5	2	2	0
Weight training	1	1	0	1	0

[1] 1972-1973 survey conducted by the Opinion Research Corporation for the President's Council on Physical Fitness and Sports.

The information in Table 16 represents the actual activity habits of the American population. How do these habits compare with an opinion survey conducted by the President's Council on Physical Fitness and Sports (1978) of seven highly qualified medical experts in the field of physical fitness? The results of this survey are presented in Table 17. These seven medical experts were asked to rate 14 different forms of activity, which included sport and recreational activities as well as conditioning-type activities. The activities were evaluated with respect to their contribution to factors of physical fitness as well as to factors of general well-being, and a total score or rating was derived for each of the 14 activities. Comparing the two surveys, one looking at actual activity patterns and the other looking at the most desirable activity patterns, it is interesting to see that of the 55% of our adult American population who exercise, few of them are involved in those activities which will give them the greatest benefits. A 1979 Harris Poll conducted for the Perrier Company on the exercise habits of Americans indicated that only 15% of the adult population were engaged regularly in vigorous physical exercise, which was defined as expending 1,500 calories per week in sports and athletic activity, for example, jogging 15 miles per week.

It is apparent that the American population wants to be more active physically. Several recent national polls or surveys have confirmed the trend toward greater participation. There does appear to be a need, however, to redirect this renewed interest in developing an active life-style into activities that will provide a higher yield. Obviously, it would be a mistake to force people out of an activity they enjoy and into another activity which will provide improved fitness and more health-related benefits if the latter activity is one which they will never enjoy. While the best health and fitness-promoting activities are the ones which should be recommended, moderate- or low-level activities are to be preferred to no activity at all. Providing people with the basic facts as to the relative benefits of various sports and recreational activities will enable them to continue to select an activity or activities which they feel will provide them with the fun and enjoyment they

Table 17   The Ranking of 14 Sports and Exercises By Seven Medical Experts[1,2]

Factors	Jogging	Bicycling	Swimming	Skating (Ice and Roller)	Handball Squash	Nordic Skiing	Alpine Skiing	Basketball	Tennis	Calisthenics	Walking	Golf	Softball	Bowling
PHYSICAL FITNESS														
Cardiorespiratory endurance	21	19	21	18	19	19	16	19	16	10	13	8	6	5
Muscular endurance	20	18	20	17	18	19	18	17	16	13	14	8	8	5
Strength	17	16	14	15	15	15	15	15	14	16	11	9	7	5
Flexibility	9	9	15	13	16	14	14	13	14	19	7	8	9	7
Balance	17	18	12	20	17	16	21	16	16	15	8	8	7	6
GENERAL WELL-BEING														
Weight control	21	20	15	17	19	17	15	19	16	12	13	6	7	5
Muscle definition	14	15	14	14	11	12	14	13	13	18	11	6	5	5
Digestion	13	12	13	11	13	12	9	10	12	11	11	7	8	7
Sleep	16	15	16	15	12	15	12	12	11	12	14	6	7	6
Total	148	142	140	140	140	139	134	134	128	126	102	66	64	51

[1]From a survey conducted by the President's Council on Physical Fitness and Sports.
[2]Each of the seven experts rated each activity for each component on a 0-3 scale, with 0 indicating no benefit and 3 indicating maximum benefit. A cumulative rating for any 1 component of 21 indicates maximum benefit is provided by that activity.

are seeking from an exercise program, and to weigh that decision against the potential benefits to be gained from those activities.

Selecting the Appropriate Activities

There are many factors which must be considered when selecting a specific activity from the various sport and recreational activities. The following are of particular importance.

1. As has been repeatedly mentioned, the activity must be one which can be enjoyed and which holds the potential for maintaining your interest and enthusiasm over a period of years.

2. The activity must be one which can be performed conveniently in the local neighborhood or within a short distance of your job. Obviously, certain activities are not appropriate for certain regions, such as skin diving and water skiing for desert residents, or snow skiing for residents of tropical areas. Likewise, it is unwise to begin an activity where the closest facility is a 30-minute commute across town. Exercise facilities and equipment must be reasonably accessible, or your personal exercise program will not have a very good chance of survival. To be beneficial, the activity must be pursued at least twice a week, and even more frequently if possible. Driving long distances, having to wait in line to use a facility, and the unavailability of an appropriate shower and dressing facility are certainly undesirable and frequently lead people to abandon their exercise programs.

3. The expense of participating in an activity must be considered. Almost any activity will have some associated costs. These costs will vary considerably, from a $40 to $50 pair of running shoes for the jogger, to several hundred dollars or more for the downhill skier. It is advisable to seek out an experienced participant in an ac-

tivity to determine what the average yearly cost will be. For some activities, the "hidden costs" are substantial, such as in boating.

4.   Select an activity that doesn't require assembling 18 or 22 bodies, such as baseball and football!

Since the focus of this book is on the promotion of improvement in health and fitness, the final, but most important, consideration should be the health and fitness benefit derived from participation in the activity. Professor Leroy "Bud" Getchell (1979) of Indiana University has attempted to classify the various recreational and sport activities on the basis of their appropriateness for developing cardiorespiratory fitness, strength, muscular endurance, and flexibility. Table 18 summarizes this general classification and expands on the information provided in Table 17. From both Tables 17 and 18, the relative merits of most popular sports and recreational activities are clearly presented. However, there are certainly exceptions to these ratings. The level of playing ability will definitely influence the benefit to be gained from an activity, as will the intensity of effort. While handball may rate as a good all-around conditioning activity, if the person does not have the skill level necessary, or doesn't pursue the sport vigorously, few benefits will result. The information provided in these two tables assumes that the participants have the skill level and motivation to achieve the maximum benefits from that exercise, and in addition these tables are intended only as a guide. Table 19 provides the relative metabolic costs of many activities.

Table 18   The Development of Specific Physical Fitness Components Through Various Sports and Recreational Activities[1]

Continuous Cardiorespiratory Endurance	Intermittent Cardiorespiratory Fitness	Strength	Muscular Endurance	Flexibility
Bicycling	Badminton	Calisthenics	Calisthenics	Calisthenics
Canoeing	Dancing	Canoeing	Canoeing	Modern dance
Cross-country skiing	Gymnastics	Cycling	Cycling	Fencing
Jogging/running	Handball	Modern dance	Modern dance	Gymnastics
Orienteering	Ice skating	Fencing	Gymnastics	Handball
Skin/scuba diving	Jog-walk-jog	Gymnastics	Handball	Ice skating
Swimming	Racquetball/handball	Hiking	Hiking	Judo
	Surfing	Ice skating	Ice skating	Karate
	Tennis	Judo	Jogging/running	Skin diving
		Karate	Judo	
		Skiing	Karate	

(Cont.)

Table 18 (Cont.)

Continuous Cardiorespiratory Endurance	Intermittent Cardiorespiratory Fitness	Strength	Muscular Endurance	Flexibility
		Racquetball/ handball	Orienteering	Skiing
		Surfing	Skin/scuba diving	Racquetball/ handball
		Strength training	Skiing	Strength training
		Swimming	Strength training	Surfing
		Water skiing	Surfing	Swimming
			Swimming	Tennis
			Tennis	Water skiing
			Water skiing	

[1]Adapted from Getchell, B. (1979). *Physical fitness: A way of life* (2nd ed.). New York: John Wiley.

Table 19   Selected Activities and Their Respective MET Values[1]

SELF-CARE ACTIVITIES	METS
Rest, supine	1.0
Sitting	1.0
Standing, relaxed	1.0
Eating	1.0
Conversation	1.0
Dressing and undressing	2.0
Washing hands and face	2.0
Propulsion, wheelchair	2.0
Walking, 2.5 m.p.h.	3.0
Showering	3.5
Walking down stairs	4.5
Walking, 3.5 m.p.h.	5.5
Ambulation, braces and crutches	6.5

HOUSEWORK ACTIVITIES	
Handsewing	1.0
Sweeping floor	1.5
Machine sewing	1.5
Polishing furniture	2.0
Peeling potatoes	2.5
Scrubbing, standing	2.5
Washing small clothes	2.5
Kneading dough	2.5
Scrubbing floors	3.0
Cleaning windows	3.0
Making beds	3.0
Ironing, standing	3.5
Mopping	3.5
Wringing wash by hand	3.5
Hanging wash	3.5
Beating carpets	4.0

OCCUPATIONAL ACTIVITIES	
Sitting at desk	1.5
Writing	1.5
Riding in automobile	1.5
Watch repairing	1.5
Typing	2.0
Welding	2.5
Radio assembly	2.5
Playing musical instrument	2.5

(Cont.)

Table 19   (cont.)

OCCUPATIONAL ACTIVITIES (cont.)

Parts assembly	3.0
Bricklaying and plastering	3.5
Heavy assembly work	4.0
Wheeling wheelbarrow 115 lb., 2.5 m.p.h.	4.0
Carpentry	5.5
Mowing lawn by handmower	6.5
Chopping wood	6.5
Shoveling	7.0
Digging	7.5

PHYSICAL-CONDITIONING ACTIVITIES

Level walking, 2 m.p.h. (1 mi. in 30 min.)	2.5
Level cycling, 5.5 m.p.h. (1 mi. in 10 min. 54 sec.)	3.0
Level cycling, 6 m.p.h. (1 mi. in 10 min.)	3.5
Level walking 2.5 m.p.h. (1 mi. in 24 min.)	3.5
Level walking, 3 m.p.h. (1 mi. in 20 min.)	4.5
Calisthenics	4.5
Level cycling, 9.7 m.p.h. (1 mi. in 6 min. 18 sec.)	5.0
Swimming, crawl, 1 ft./sec.	5.0
Level walking, 3.5 m.p.h. (1 mi. in 17 min.)	5.5
Level walking, 4.0 m.p.h. (1 mi. in 15 min.)	6.5
Level jogging, 5.0 m.p.h. (1 mi. in 12 min.)	7.5
Level cycling, 13 m.p.h. (1 mi. in 4 min. 37 sec.)	9.0
Level running, 7.5 m.p.h. (1 mi. in 8 min.)	9.0
Swimming, crawl, 2 ft./sec.	10.0
Level running, 8.5 m.p.h. (1 mi. in 7 min.)	12.0
Level running, 10.0 m.p.h. (1 mi. in 6 min.)	15.0
Swimming, crawl, 2.5 ft./sec.	15.0
Swimming, crawl, 3.0 ft./sec.	20.0
Level running, 12 m.p.h. (1 mi. in 5 min.)	20.0
Level running, 15 m.p.h. (¼ mi. in 1 min.)	30.0
Swimming, crawl, 3.5 ft./sec.	30.0

(Cont.)

Table 19   (cont.)

RECREATIONAL ACTIVITIES

Painting, sitting	1.5
Playing piano	2.0
Driving car	2.0
Canoeing, 2.5 m.p.h.	2.5
Horseback riding, walk	2.5
Volleyball, 6-man recreational	3.0
Billiards	3.0
Bowling	3.5
Horseshoes	3.5
Golf	4.0
Cricket	4.0
Archery	4.5
Ballroom dancing	4.5
Table tennis	4.5
Baseball	4.5
Tennis	6.0
Horseback riding, trot	6.5
Folk dancing	6.5
Skiing	8.0
Horseback riding, gallop	8.0
Squash rackets	8.5
Fencing	9.0
Basketball	9.0
Football	9.0
Gymnastics	10.0
Handball and paddleball	10.0

[1]Adapted from Wilmore, J.H. (1982). *Training for sport and activity*. (2nd ed.). Boston: Allyn and Bacon.

Competition

It is fascinating to observe the phenomenal increase in young, middle-aged, and older adults who have turned to competition as an outgrowth or extension of their exercise program. Many individuals who took up racquetball as a recreational sport are now entering tournaments both at their local club and at other clubs in the community, and enjoying the excitement of competition. Recreational joggers are turning to road races, and a growing number are increasing their training mileage and intensity with the hope of one day conquering the full 26.2-mile marathon. The record number of participants competing in marathons in the late 1970s and early 1980s attests to this fact. While a field of 100 runners was considered a big marathon in the early 1970s, there are 10,000 or more entering a number of the more popular marathons in the 1980s! Master's and Senior's competition has become extremely popular in swimming and track and field. These programs provide formal, high-level competitive experiences for men and women 30 years of age and over, with competition broken down into either 5- or 10-year increments. Official world records are kept, and there are yearly national and international meets in addition to numerous state and local meets.

Is such competition advisable? The answer to that question is a qualified yes. If the individual has been medically cleared for competition, and has been properly trained for his or her specific event, then competition can provide enjoyable experiences and will be a good motivator for maintaining high levels of fitness. One can't help but be caught up in the excitement and enthusiasm when watching these older athletes compete. The smiles on their faces, the appearance of their lean and healthy bodies, and the tremendous performances they are able to achieve are all indications of the positive nature of competition. However, some of these competitors fail to obtain proper medical clearance, and/or don't properly train for competition, and the result has been unfortunate for some, and even fatal for others. Several heart attacks have occurred either during or immediately following competition. Too often, the sprinter is the one who fails to properly train, for speed is such a natural or genetic factor. A sprinter can maintain a certain amount of speed without maintaining good physical condition. An overweight, 3-pack-a-day smoker with high blood pressure is a likely candidate for serious cardiovascular complications from burst-type physical activity, even though that person may still possess relatively good speed. Proper conditioning, preceded by an appropriate medical clearance, is essential for safe participation in competition.

How do you properly train for competition? For those in sports such as racquetball, handball, and tennis, a good fitness foundation is essential, but once that has been established it is imperative that the focus be on skill improvement. To have an outstanding level of fitness without a high level of skill will win few, if any, matches! When the appropriate conditioning level has been achieved, the serious competitor in skill activities must begin working on the fine points of the game, including hours of practice to develop the appropriate techniques, coordination, and sense or feeling of where to be on the court or field. Strategy must also be a major consideration. In short, for those in skill activities, they must become students of their game. The higher up the competition ladder they climb, the more meaningful are the subtle, small points of the game. There are many excellent books which have been written specifically for the serious competitor in most of the currently popular sports for additional information relative to the fine points of a sport or activity.

For the serious runner, cyclist, or swimmer, skill is an important factor, but even more important is the level of training or conditioning. The competitive runner, cyclist, or swimmer must have a highly structured training program which will provide the means to accomplish a specific goal. The information in Tables 20 and 21 was prepared for competitive runners. However, it can also be applied to competitive cyclists and competitive swimmers. In Table 20, the swimmer can approximate training requirements by dividing the distance under the column "Event" by 4, using these new distances as a guide. The cyclist should multiply these dis-

Table 20   Training Requirements for Various Running Distances[1]

Event	Aerobic	Anaerobic/Speed
Ultramarathon	100	0
Marathon	90	10
15,000 meters (9.3 miles)	85	15
10,000 meters (6.2 miles)	80	20
5,000 meters (3.1 miles)	70	30
3,000 meters ($\approx$2 miles)	45	55
1,500 meters ($\approx$1 mile)	40	60
800 meters ($\approx$½ mile)	30	70
400 meters ($\approx$440 yards)	20	80
200 meters ($\approx$220 yards)	10	90
100 meters ($\approx$100 yards)	5	95

[1]The figures in this table represent the percentage of emphasis in training. These percentages will change depending on whether the athlete is in-season or out-of-season.

Table 21   Components of Various Systems of Endurance and Sprint Training

Type of Training	Aerobic	Anaerobic/Speed
Interval training		
Short intervals (100-200 meters)	low	high
Medium intervals (400-800 meters)	moderate	high
Long intervals (greater than 800 meters)	high	moderate
Continuous training		
High intensity	high	moderate
Low intensity (LSD)	high	low
Fartlek	high	moderate

tances by a factor of 2 or 3. Again, as with the highly skilled athlete in game-type activities, the competitive runner, cyclist, and swimmer are referred to any one of a number of excellent books and magazines which provide much more detail on the design of training programs as well as racing strategies.

Special Considerations Related to Exercise and Sport

From the novice who has just made the commitment to start an exercise program to the elite athlete, there are many aspects of conditioning and competition which must be understood in order to have a safe, profitable, and enjoyable experience. The environment presents many unique challenges which must be faced intelligently, or the individual risks the possibility of serious injury. Heat, humidity, direct radiation from the sun, cold, altitude, and air pollution are the major factors that will influence the individual during exercise or competition. Understanding the problems associated with and learning effective methods for coping with these environmental stresses will be the focus of chapter 9. Differences in the responses to exercise and athletic competition between the sexes and with age will be discussed in chapter 10. Chapter 11 will outline nutritional requirements for healthy living and discuss whether nutritional supplements actually facilitate or improve athletic performance. The final chapter, chapter 12, will review the myriad of injuries which can result from sport and activity and discuss the various alternatives for effectively treating these injuries, in addition to ways of preventing injury.

Environmental Factors

It is a well-known fact that, in certain sports or events, the performance of the athlete will depend to a large extent on the environment. The winning time in the Boston Marathon can vary by as much as 10 minutes or more, depending on whether the race is performed under conditions of 44° F and a light rain, or 92° F, high humidity, and no cloud cover, which are actual extremes which runners have faced in Boston over the years. A basketball team that trains and practices at sea level is suddenly transported to an altitude of 7,000 feet and finds that their typical fast-break offense and pressing-zone defense fall apart because the players are literally exhausted. Some sports or activities are not influenced to a great extent by the environment, since they are played or performed in a sheltered environment, altitude excluded. Wrestlers, gymnasts, and swimmers are seldom influenced by the environment since they are either performing indoors in a highly controlled environment, or outdoors in a pool which is also highly controlled with respect to temperature and humidity. A sport such as football can place extreme environmental stresses on its athletes, with pre-season practice beginning in July or August and competition ending in November, December, or January, depending on the level of competition, high school, college, or professional. During the time span of the football season, these athletes are exposed to the extremes of heat and humidity in most regions of the United States in the early part of the season, and the bitter cold, ice, and snow at season's end.

While the above examples are oriented toward the high-performance or elite athlete, the recreational athlete and the individual who is exercising for improved health must contend with these same problems. This chapter will briefly outline the problems associated with exercising under various environmental conditions, and will then discuss how one can effectively contend with each of these stresses.

Variations in Temperature and Humidity

The body is not a very efficient engine. For all of the fuel it uses, only a small percentage of this fuel is translated into useful work. The efficiency of performing various exercises or activities varies considerably, from less than 10% for swimming, to 20% or greater for walking, jogging, or bicycling. The energy that is required by the body to produce work is expended in the ratio of approximately 15% to 25% for the actual work produced, and 75% to 85% lost due to inefficiency in the form of heat, which amounts to approximately 80 kilocalories per hour of excess heat at rest and up to 900 kilocalories per hour or more during exhaustive exercise. This is illustrated by the increased warmth one feels when exercising on a cool day, or the extreme heat stress when exercising on a hot day. The amount of heat produced by the body during exercise is considerable. In cold weather, this increased body heat is welcomed. In warm environments, this increased body heat can be fatal.

As the body starts to exercise, the metabolic rate increases in direct proportion to the intensity of exercise, as does the additional heat which is generated from the body's inefficient utilization of its energy. Since body temperature must be very carefully controlled, there is a critical need to rid the body of this increasing internal heat load. The major adjustment made by the body to promote heat loss is the redirection or shunting of warm blood from the central core of the body to the periphery or skin, as evidenced by the red skin of an overheated athlete. When blood is brought to the body's surface, this allows heat to be lost more efficiently by *convection* and *radiation*. In convection, heat is lost or transferred from the body to a moving liquid or gas, such as cool air, while radiation involves the passing of heat from the body to the environment through electromagnetic waves. Body heat is also lost through *conduction*, or the passing of heat directly from the body to a cooler object, and *evaporation*, whereby the body sweats and the resulting water droplets are converted into water vapor. When sweat evaporates, there is a net loss of body heat which cools the surrounding skin. With the evaporation of every liter of water, there is a net loss of 580 kilocalories of heat.

Body Temperature Regulation

Body temperature is controlled by a small area in the very center of the brain referred to as the hypothalamus. The adjacent pre-optic area of the brain and special temperature sensors in the skin are also involved in temperature control. At rest, body temperature is regulated to a very constant value of 98.6° F, although the actual temperature at which this control is established will vary from one individual to the next. With exercise, the body readjusts its thermostat, allowing the temperature to increase to temperatures in excess of 100° F, and in prolonged exhaustive exercise to temperatures that can exceed 106° F. The resetting of the body's thermostat to allow higher body temperatures during exercise appears to be a desirable alteration, as the chemical reactions for energy production and the availability of oxygen are enhanced or facilitated at these higher temperatures.

Exercise in the Heat

When exercising in the heat, the effective heat stress is determined by the temperature, humidity, radiation from the sun, air movement, the intensity and duration of the exercise, and acclimatization, which depends on the extent of previous exposure to similar environmental conditions. The fluid and mineral intake both before and during exercise is also an important factor.

High Temperature.   When the temperature of the surrounding environment equals or exceeds the temperature of the skin (92° F to 93° F), convection, conduction, and radiation are no longer effective avenues of heat loss, and can actually become avenues of heat gain when the surrounding temperature exceeds the skin temperature. At this point, the body must rely totally on evaporation for heat loss. This works well for the individual exercising in hot, dry environments, but in hot, humid environments, the surrounding air is already highly saturated with water vapor, which limits the amount of sweat that can be evaporated. The higher the humidity, the lower will be the volume of available sweat that will be evaporated. In a hot, dry environment, the individual isn't even aware of the fact that he or she is sweating, because the sweat is evaporated just as soon as it reaches the skin. As the humidity increases, there is a decrease in the volume of sweat evaporated and the individual is suddenly aware of the fact that he or she is sweating. When the body's regulatory mechanisms fail or when the environmental stresses are such that the body can no longer effectively lose body heat, the individual is placed in a potentially lethal situation.

As the environmental temperature increases, there is a smaller temperature gradient between the body and the surrounding air. This increases the reliance on evaporation, and, in fact, evaporation can become the only avenue of heat loss, as was described above, once the surrounding temperature exceeds the skin temperature. Evaporation requires sweating, so with an increased reliance on evaporation, there is an increased demand for sweating. Since the fluid lost through sweating comes primarily from the plasma volume of the blood, the total blood volume is reduced, imposing an even greater demand on the cardiovascular system. As the environmental temperature continues to rise, more blood is redirected to the periphery in an attempt to increase the cooling of the body's central core, while the rate of sweating continues to increase, further reducing the blood volume. With a reduced blood volume resulting from increased sweating, and a reduced central blood volume due to a redirection of the blood to the periphery, the total volume of blood available to serve the active muscles is greatly reduced, and the performance of the individual is greatly restricted. Most individuals are well aware of the fact that they just can't perform the same quality or quantity of work when they must exercise in the heat. In long-distance runners, the sweat loss may approach 6% to 10% of the runner's body weight. We are capable of sweating up to 2 liters or more per hour. Up to an 18% reduction in plasma volume has been found in exercise with losses of 4% of the total body weight.

Humidity, Air Velocity, and Radiation.   It is clear that environmental temperature alone is not an accurate index of the total physiological stress experienced by the individual during exercise. Humidity is an extremely important factor, for dry air is necessary for efficient evaporation to occur, and evaporation is the major avenue of heat loss. Air velocity is also an important factor, since the movement of air is necessary to continuously replenish the air surrounding the body. With a low air velocity, the air surrounding the body becomes saturated with water, and this restricts the efficient evaporation of sweat. The degree of cloud cover also influences the degree of physiological stress. Without cloud cover, direct radiation from the sun adds considerably to the total heat stress. Full or partial cloud cover provides tremendous relief when exercising in the heat.

Dehydration.   One of the major problems associated with exercise in the heat is the resulting dehydration. As was stated above, up to 2 liters of sweat per hour or more can be lost during prolonged exhaustive exercise in the heat, which would be the equivalent of nearly 5 pounds per hour of weight loss. Marathon runners will typically lose 5 to 7 pounds during the course of the 26.2-mile race even though they drink freely during the race. Along with water, salts and other essential electrolytes are lost at a substantial rate. With the loss of every 1% of body weight, there is an estimated increase of 0.3° F to 0.5° F in body temperature. Obviously, everything possible should be done to decrease the rate of dehydration, since extreme dehydration has serious consequences which will be discussed later.

An essential part of any measure taken to prevent dehydration is to provide abundant fluids for the individual before, during, and following the activity. At one time, it was considered dangerous for athletes to consume fluids during practices or games. It was feared that fluid ingestion would cause severe cramping of the stomach and the intestine, so all fluids were generally withheld until after the practice or competition. It is now recognized that the practice of withholding water was the worst course of action that could be taken. Liberal ingestion of fluids during exercise is essential whenever dehydration is a potential problem. Fluid ingestion both before and during exercise has been shown to reduce the increase in rectal temperature as exercise is prolonged for up to 2 hours. For the same level of work and thermal stress, exercise with fluid ingestion results in a deep body temperature that is approximately 1.5° F lower when compared to the same situation with no fluid. One additional fact that has an important bearing on dehydration: we do not voluntarily drink enough fluid to replace that which is lost. As a result, the individual should be encouraged to drink as much as possible both before and during the exercise period. Fluid breaks during exercise are to be strongly encouraged.

What type of fluid should be consumed before and during exercise? Water is readily available and cheap, but there have been major advertising campaigns and testimonials which encourage the consumption of specially formulated electrolyte solutions, and some are now promoting the use of beer as a fluid replacement drink. The most appropriate fluid replacement drink may, in fact, be water. Most of the presently available commercial drinks have too high a sugar content, and as the concentration of sugar in a drink is increased, its rate of emptying from the stomach is decreased. The most critical factor in fluid replacement is to get the water out of the stomach and into the blood. The water replacement function of a fluid replacement drink is much more essential than that of electrolyte replacement, or providing glucose or sugar to the body for activities of up to 3 or 4 hours duration. Professor Carl Gisolfi of the University of Iowa has made several suggestions relative to fluid replacement that are soundly based on research. In addition to drinking liberal amounts of fluid prior to exercise, he recommends drinking approximately one-half of a pint of a glucose-electrolyte solution every 15 to 20 minutes during exercise. The glucose content of the solution should be less than 2.5 grams for every 100 milliliters of solution. The solution should be cool, slightly hypotonic, and palatable to the individual. Lastly, he suggests that a liberal salting of foods at mealtime will be sufficient to replace the salt which was lost through sweating during and following exercise.

Heat Disorders.   One of the major problems associated with dehydration is the potential for heat disorders. When the body is unable to successfully adapt to thermal stress, there are three forms of failure which can result. *Heat cramps* is the least serious of the three, and is the direct result of the salt and water loss with dehydration. It is characterized by severe cramping of the skeletal muscles. *Heat exhaustion* is the next most serious heat disorder, and is characterized by body temperatures of from 101° F to 104° F, extreme tiredness, breathlessness, dizziness, and a rapid pulse. These symptoms are probably the result of a reduced sweat production, indicating the initial failure of the body's ability to effectively cope with the heat stress. *Heat stroke* is the most serious of the three forms of heat disorder, and is characterized by body temperatures of

105° F or higher, cessation of sweating, total confusion, and eventual unconsciousness. The victim of heat stroke will likely die if left untreated. When heat stroke occurs, extreme measures have to be taken to cool the body, such as immersion in cold water.

While the above discussion might lead one to totally abandon all unnecessary forms of activity when the environmental temperatures start to climb, it should be emphasized that exercise during the hot-weather months can be performed with minimal risk, providing certain precautionary measures are taken.

1. Exercise should not be performed during the hottest part of the day in the direct sun. Early morning and/or early or mid-evening are the most desirable times to exercise since the direct radiation from the sun can be avoided and it is typically cooler at those times.

2. Wear the appropriate attire, which, in the heat, simply means to wear as little as one can legally get away with. For males, a light pair of shorts, brief socks, and shoes are ideal, and females can simply add a brief halter top. The more clothing that is in contact with the skin's surface, the more evaporation will be restricted, and the heat stress increased. Clothing should be loose-weaved and light in color to reflect heat. Under no conditions, even in the middle of winter, should one wear a rubberized suit. This has become a popular way to lose weight, but it is an extremely dangerous procedure, and the weight loss, while substantial, is all water loss, which is regained within the subsequent 24 hours. Within a short period of time, the air within the rubberized suit becomes fully saturated with water vapor. Since the temperature inside the suit exceeds the skin temperature, and usually exceeds the deep body temperature, with the air totally saturated, all avenues of heat loss are lost and the result is a steady increase in body temperature. The combination of profuse sweating and a rapidly increasing body temperature makes the individual who wears the rubberized suit particularly vulnerable to heat disorders.

3. Drink liberally prior to starting to exercise, and plan to stop every 10 to 15 minutes for water, or some other acceptable fluid replacement solution.
4. Do not exercise when the temperature exceeds 90° F to 95° F, and this recommendation should be reduced accordingly when the humidity exceeds 40% to 50%. The intensity and duration of exercise can also be reduced at temperatures below 90° F.
5. Always stay aware of the symptoms of the three heat disorders, and stop exercising when any symptoms start to appear. One symptom which was not mentioned earlier, but which is an extremely important one, is the sudden feeling of being chilled, including the appearance of "goose bumps," or piloerection. When this occurs, the sweating mechanism is starting to fail and the body temperature is being reset to a higher level, which could lead directly to heat stroke.

One additional precaution that can be taken to reduce the risk of exercising in hot weather is to become gradually adapted to the heat stress, a process which is referred to as acclimatization. Repeated exposure to the stress of heat results in a general adaptation which enables the body to better tolerate additional heat stress. While acclimatization will not enable the body to perform maximally under extremes in heat as it could under normal temperatures, it does enable the body to perform the same levels of work more efficiently in the heat, and allows the performance of even higher levels of work before the temperature regulating system fails. Total, or nearly total, acclimatization can occur within a 5- to 14-day period.

Exercise in the Cold

When compared to the potential problems of exercise in the heat, exercise in the cold presents relatively few problems. As with heat, cold stress is the result of factors other than just environmental temperature. The wind creates a chill factor, and the more moist the surrounding air, the greater the phys-

Table 22 Wind Chill Factor Chart¹,²

Estimated Wind Speed (in m.p.h.)	Actual Thermometer Reading (°F)											
	50	40	30	20	10	0	-10	-20	-30	-40	-50	-60
	Equivalent Temperature (°F)											
calm	50	40	30	20	10	0	-10	-20	-30	-40	-50	-60
5	48	37	27	16	6	-5	-15	-26	-36	-47	-57	-68
10	40	28	16	4	-9	-24	-33	-46	-58	-70	-83	-95
15	36	22	9	-5	-18	-32	-45	-58	-72	-85	-99	-112
20	32	18	4	-10	-25	-39	-53	-67	-82	-96	-110	-124
25	30	16	0	-15	-29	-44	-59	-74	-88	-104	-118	-133
30	28	13	-2	-18	-33	-48	-63	-79	-94	-109	-125	-140
35	27	11	-4	-20	-35	-51	-67	-82	-98	-113	-129	-145
40	26	10	-6	-21	-37	-53	-69	-85	-100	-116	-132	-148
(Wind speeds greater than 40 m.p.h. have little additional effect)	Green				Yellow			Red			Great Danger	

Little Danger (for properly clothed person); maximum danger of false sense of security

Increasing Danger Danger from freezing of exposed flesh

Great Danger

¹Adapted from *Runner's World* (1973). **8**, 28.
²Trenchfoot and immersion foot may occur at any point on this chart.

iologic stress. A dry, still day at 10° F in the direct sun is much more tolerable than a moist, windy day at 40° F with complete cloud cover. *Runner's World* magazine published an article in 1973 which provided sound guidelines for exercising in the cold. These guidelines are summarized in Table 22.

The clothing worn while exercising in the cold is very important. First, there is a tendency to overdress. It must be remembered that exercise will, by itself, create a considerable amount of heat. This can lead to profuse sweating if the person has overdressed. Sweat-soaked clothing in a cold, dry climate will lead to rapid evaporation with the resulting loss of body heat, which then can lead to severe chilling. Clothing should be put on in layers, and as the body starts to warm naturally as a result of the increased body heat accompanying exercise, the outer layers of clothing should be removed as necessary to prevent overheating and excessive sweating. Tightly woven garments will help to maintain a small pocket of warm moist air between the skin and the garment. Thermal underwear is recommended for the arms, legs, and torso in extreme cold, and gloves and a double pair of socks are also helpful. Since a great deal of body heat is lost through the head, a stocking cap or some other form of appropriate headwear would be most important. Males may wish to wear an additional pair of shorts or a pair of cotton briefs to protect their genitalia, since frostbite of the penis has been reported on a number of occasions, with the rather humorous documentation of one celebrated case in the prestigious *New England Journal of Medicine*.

Altitude

As altitude increases, total air pressure decreases, as does the partial pressure of oxygen. As a result, increases in altitude (above 7,000 feet) will cause a reduction in both the amount of oxygen carried in the arterial blood and the amount of oxygen that is transferred from the blood into the cell. This limits the availability of oxygen and reduces maximal oxygen uptake, limiting physical working capacity in direct proportion to the increase in altitude. Simply stated, there is less oxygen available to the body's tissues. Activities of short duration are influenced little, if any, by altitude. In fact, certain activities, such as the long jump or sprints, may actually be enhanced by altitude, due to the thinner or less dense air providing less resistance while the body is in flight. Activities of a longer duration are definitely influenced by increases in altitude. It appears that the greater the aerobic component, the more the activity will be negatively influenced by altitude, and the higher the altitude, the greater the decrement in performance.

Can one adapt or acclimatize to altitude in the same way that one can acclimatize to heat? The body does acclimatize to a certain extent, but this acclimatization is never sufficient to allow athletic performance to duplicate that found at sea level. A major change that takes place during the initial few hours at altitude is an increase in the number of red blood cells, which is the body's way of adapting to the limitations in the delivery of oxygen to the cell. There is also a substantial loss in plasma volume which is the result of acute dehydration. Within a week to 10 days the plasma volume returns to near-normal levels. With the increase in red blood cells comes an increase in hemoglobin, and this facilitates oxygen delivery to the tissues. Maximal oxygen uptake is reduced substantially when first arriving at altitude, but it begins to increase with the increase in red blood cells and hemoglobin. This last response to altitude has led researchers, coaches, and athletes to postulate that high-altitude training might provide certain advantages to the athlete on return to sea level. Supposedly, every gold medal winner in the 1972 Munich Olympic Games running events from the 1,500 meters through the marathon were altitude trained. While a logical case can be made for altitude training physiologically, those few studies which have been conducted lend little or no support to this theory.

For the competitive athlete, recreational athlete, or the individual who is exercising for its health-related benefits, brief sojourns to altitudes above 5,000 feet will result in decreases in the ability to perform aerobic-type activities. Recognizing this, adjust your workout or pace in competition accordingly, with the understanding that both intensity and duration will by necessity be reduced.

Air Pollution

Scientists have become quite concerned about the possible problems that might be experienced while exercising in an environment where there is a high level of air pollution. The air in most cities is contaminated with small particles and gases that present serious health problems when present in large concentrations. When air becomes stagnant or when a temperature inversion occurs, some of these air pollutants reach levels of concentration that produce significant detrimental effects on athletic performance. Carbon monoxide, photochemical oxidants, and sulfur oxides are the major contaminants.

Carbon monoxide is an odorless gas that has a high affinity for the blood's hemoglobin. As carbon monoxide levels increase, the red blood cells become increasingly bound to carbon monoxide and lose their ability to transport oxygen. Both maximal and submaximal performance become limited once blood levels of carbon monoxide reach certain critical levels. Ozone, the primary photochemical oxidant, causes severe irritation of the eyes and chest, and breathlessness, coughing and nausea are the primary complaints. Ozone can also limit your maximal and submaximal performance once certain critical levels are attained. Sulfur dioxide is the major sulfur oxide contaminant. It acts as a lung irritant during exercise and can limit performance.

To avoid problems of exercising in an environment with high levels of air pollution, you should not exercise during those times when traffic is heavy, when the the temperature and humidity are elevated, or when smog alerts have been issued.

10

Sex and Aging

Over the years, it has become traditional to refer to females as the weaker sex. During the 1970s, in the United States, the range of roles and career opportunities available to women was greatly expanded. The 1970s observed the emergence of the female athlete. Where the athletic arena had traditionally been the domain of the male, females were now demanding equal opportunities, including budgets, coaching, facilities, equipment, and competitive opportunities. With the gain in popularity and support of women's sports came a tremendous improvement in national and world records. Girls and women were beginning to close the gap between their records and those of the boys and men. On the basis of world records in the year 1985, the male was 8.4% faster in the 100-meter dash; jumped 14.0% higher in the high jump; ran 11.0% faster in the 1,500-meter run; and swam 7.5% faster in the 400-meter free-style swim. These are very impressive differences and tend to point to continued male superiority and dominance until a further check of the record books indicates that in 1976, East Germany's 15-year-old Petra Thümer swam the 400-meter free-style in what was then a women's world record time of 4:09.9, just slightly less than 3 seconds faster than

Don Schollander's world record time of 4:12.2 in the 1964 Olympic Games. In analyzing the past records for the 400-meter free-style, Dr. Ernst Jokl has predicted that by sometime in the 1990s, the women will be swimming this distance as fast as men! Are women truly the weaker sex—biologically inferior—or do these differences in athletic performance reflect past social and cultural restrictions? This question, and other questions dealing with the female in exercise and sport and the influence of age on exercise and sport performance, will be covered in this chapter.

The Female in Exercise and Sport

At full maturity, the average female is 5 inches shorter than the average male, 30 to 40 pounds lighter in total weight, 40 to 50 pounds lighter in lean body weight, and is considerably fatter, 25% versus 15% body fat. Up to the time of puberty, however, the average female is equal or greater in both height and weight, which is probably the result of the earlier maturation patterns of the female. At maturity, the male is characterized by broader shoulders, narrower hips, and a greater chest girth relative to his total size. These differences are due, at least in part, to the influence of the predominant sex hormones which begin to have their impact at puberty. The predominantly male sex hormone, testosterone, promotes the growth of the lean tissue, having a major effect on increasing the muscle mass. Estrogen, the predominantly female sex hormone, promotes the deposition of fat. The mature female has higher amounts of essential, sex-specific fat in the breasts and other areas of the body. Thus, the female appears destined to have substantially more body fat and less muscle mass than her male counterpart, which would put her at a distinct disadvantage in the performance of most athletic events. Is this necessarily true, or are there other factors which haven't been considered?

Body Composition

The average female at full maturity (18 to 22 years of age) will have between 22% and 26% of her weight as body fat. The average male of similar age will have a body composition of only 12% to 16% body fat. However, when one looks at male and female athletes who have had similar training experience in competitive sport, the difference between the sexes is much less, particularly for those sports that have a significant aerobic or cardiorespiratory endurance component. Table 3 in the first chapter of this book provided information on the relative fat values of males and females in various sports. While the females have typically higher relative fat values for each sport, in certain sports there is an overlap in the range of values for the two sexes. In a study of 78 elite female runners, 12 had relative fat values under 10%, and nearly half were below 15%. Three of these female runners were at 6% body fat, a figure which is approximately the average for world-class male distance runners. One of those three women had started a running program because of a weight problem. She eventually reduced her weight from 148 to 118 pounds, and, in the process, at one time held the best time in the world for the women's marathon. From this study, and others, it would appear that the average female is too fat, and that she has the potential to decrease her relative body fat values to 20% or less. The female athlete should attempt to drop her relative body fat to a level of 15% or less.

The higher values seen in the "average" female, and even in some female athletes, are more than likely the result of a sedentary life-style, which is acquired shortly after she reaches puberty. The male remains considerably more active than the female during the teens and early 20s, and begins to assume a more sedentary existence shortly after he marries, at approximately 25 years of age. Interestingly, the 35-year-old male has an average relative body fat of approximately 19% to 22%. Apparently, 10 years of sedentary living takes its toll in the male in much the same way it does in the female; the assumption of a sedentary life-style just comes some 10 to 15 years later in life.

Strength, Muscular Endurance, and Flexibility

There have been numerous studies which have confirmed the well-known fact that males are stronger than females. Recently, however, several studies have indicated that the earlier observations and opinions might not be totally correct. In a study of college men and women, men were found to be considerably stronger in both lower body as well as upper body strength. When strength was related to the size of the body, the strength of the legs was essentially identical in the two sexes. In other words, the quality of the muscle appears to be similar for men and women. Given the same amount of muscle mass, the expected strength would be essentially the same. With respect to upper body strength, the women were substantially weaker, even when strength was expressed relative to body size. For a man and a woman of the same body weight, the muscle mass of the legs is quite similar, while the muscle mass of the chest, shoulders, and arms is considerably greater in the man. Thus, strength is a function of the size of the muscle, or the amount of muscle mass, and is probably not related to the sex of the individual. Sex does contribute indirectly, however, in that the female will never have the absolute body size of the male, and the muscle mass in the upper body will probably always be proportionally less in the female. In studies where muscle biopsies were obtained from men and women athletes in the same sport, the proportion of the different muscle fiber types was similar between the sexes, although the men appeared to have larger fibers.

Studies of women who have participated in strength training programs for periods of 2 to 6 months have demonstrated that women, like men, can substantially increase their basic levels of strength. In fact, women are likely to achieve greater relative gains in strength since they are typically starting at a much lower percentage of their ultimate capacity. Average increases in strength of as much as 30% have been noted following 10 weeks of weight training; however, some of the women in one particular study were able to double their strength in selected areas of the body. It appears that the female has the ability to substantially alter her basic strength in a rather short period of time. In addition, studies have shown that changes in the size of the muscles with increases in strength are considerably less in females than in males, which is undoubtedly the result of differences in the concentrations of their predominant sex hormones. This is an important point, for at one time, strength training for women was strongly discouraged for fear that those who did strength-train would develop large, bulky muscles.

There is very limited information available on the similarities or differences between males and females in muscular endurance and flexibility. Muscular endurance is typically highly related to the strength of the muscle or muscle group, and is therefore probably greater in males, although after a period of intense training there should be little, if any, difference. Traditional field tests of muscular endurance, such as maximum number of pull-ups, or sit-ups, indicate much greater levels of muscular endurance in males. These tests, however, may not be an accurate reflection of muscular endurance as an isolated, pure component; there may be factors other than muscular endurance which are causing the substantial difference between males and females. Flexibility appears to be much greater in the female at all ages. Even with considerable training, the female maintains an edge in flexibility. This is probably a genetically endowed advantage which could be the result of sex-specific hormone differences.

Cardiorespiratory Endurance Capacity

In previous chapters, and in Table 8, it was indicated that females have a lower maximal oxygen uptake capacity when compared to males, at the age of 10 to 12 years and older. Prior to 10 to 12 years of age, the values for males and females are nearly identical. Several factors have been suggested as the primary explanation for these differences. First, the female has a smaller stroke volume (volume of blood pumped per beat) than the male for the same absolute level of work, which is at least partially related to her smaller body size. In addition, hemoglobin levels in females have been reported to be lower than males of similar age by as much as 10% or more. With a smaller stroke volume at maximum work, and a similar maximum heart rate, the maximum cardiac output (volume of blood pumped per minute) will be lower in the female, and when this is combined with lower hemoglobin levels, the oxygen-carrying and oxygen-delivery capability of the female is greatly reduced. Theoretically, this explains the lower maximal oxygen uptake values in females. In studies of highly conditioned women distance runners, however, the magnitude of difference when compared to equally trained men distance runners was approximately 16%. In fact, when the best women runners were compared to the best men runners, the differences in maximal oxygen uptake were reduced to only 4.1%. From these results, it would appear that the average female has a tremendous potential for developing her cardiorespiratory endurance capacity to a level far in excess of her existing level. Optimal development of cardiorespiratory endurance capacity would be extremely beneficial for the female athlete, particularly if she is an endurance athlete.

Menstrual and Gynecological Considerations

Two questions which are foremost in the minds of many women, particularly women athletes, have to do with the influence of their menstrual cycle on athletic performance, and the influence of their training procedures and competition on menstruation and childbirth. With respect to alterations in athletic performance ability with different phases of the menstrual cycle, there appears to be a considerable amount of individual variability. Some women have absolutely no noticeable change in their ability to perform throughout the complete cycle, while other have considerable difficulty in the pre-flow and initial-flow phases of the cycle. The limited research that has been conducted tends to suggest that performance ability appears to be best in the immediate post-flow period up to the fifteenth day of the cycle, with the first day of the cycle corresponding to the initiation of the flow or menstrual phase, and with ovulation occurring on about day fourteen. The percentage of women who report impaired performance during the flow phase is approximately the same as those who experience no difficulty. In fact, some women athletes have noted their peak performance during the flow phase, including the setting of world records.

With respect to the question concerning the influence of various training procedures and intense competition on the menstrual cycle and childbirth, again, the data is very limited. Several long-term studies have been reported on former competitive swimmers, with findings that suggest that intense training at an early age has no serious consequences relative to future gynecological problems or problems with childbirth. It is generally accepted that the woman who is in excellent physical condition during pregnancy will have an easier period of labor, and fewer undesirable side effects during the actual delivery.

It is generally agreed that exercise during pregnancy is to be encouraged, not discouraged, although certain guidelines should be followed. First, the woman should discontinue exercise and consult her obstetrician if there is any unusual pain, or if there is any bleeding or rupture of membranes. She shouldn't use the initial period of pregnancy as a time to start her exercise program—she should plan in advance, if possible! She shouldn't allow her rectal or axillary (underarm) temperature to go above 101 degrees F, although this is not easily monitored in a typical social setting. Generally, she should participate in formal exercise not more than three times per week, for not longer than 30 minutes per session, and at not more than 70% of her maximal heart rate—for most, a heart rate of between 140 and 160 beats per minute would be safe. Proper nutrition, including fluids, is also important, assuring adequate intake of water, iron, calcium and vitamins, and a weight gain of 3 pounds per month, or 20 to 30 pounds total. High altitude and hot and humid weather should be avoided. Finally, exercise in the supine or back lying position should be avoided due to unfavorable decreases in blood pressure; likewise any exercise that carries any risk for abdominal trauma.

One possible problem has surfaced recently, although it is possibly not a problem but a very natural response of the body. Athletes who have trained and competed intensely in sports such as figure skating, dancing, gymnastics, cycling, and distance running have reported the absence of menses or menstrual periods for intervals of months or even years. This absence of menstrual periods or the cessation of menstruation is referred to as *secondary amenorrhea*. Oligomenorrhea, or abnormally infrequent or scanty menses, is also an associated occurrence. The actual percentage of women athletes who experience secondary amenorrhea or oligomenorrhea is not well documented, with estimates of from 4% to 12% on the low end, up to 50% on the high end. The actual percentage of women involved will probably vary according to the sport and to the intensity of training. The occurrence appears to be greater in those who are doing many hours of training each day, for example, dancers and gymnasts, and to those who are working at high intensities, such as distance runners and cyclists. Many of these athletes are thankful to be rid of the "curse," but many are also concerned about the long-term consequences. Neither the cause of secondary amenorrhea or oligomenorrhea, nor the long-term consequences are known. Some of these athletes have become pregnant during the interval of amenorrhea, which is indicative of the fact that fertility is possibly not influenced in the absence of menstruation. This latter point is an important one, for many assume that this is an effective method of birth control, and that they are safe during these intervals of cessation of menstruation. The cause may be related to low levels of weight or body fat, to the acute effects of stress, or to changes in levels of circulating hormones. Research is presently in progress to look both at cause and long-term consequences.

A major concern of women, particularly as they reach the age of menopause, is the health of their bones. While exercise has generally been considered important for optimal bone health, several recent studies have reported reductions in the mineral content of bone in women runners who are amenorrheic—a finding which has led some to seriously question whether women should be running. It has generally been accepted that exercise is important for normal bone growth and for maintaining healthy bone throughout life. In fact, in older women, several studies have indicated that those who exercise maintain, or even increase their bone mineral content, compared to a reduction in bone mineral in those who do not exercise. It has also been shown that tennis players and baseball pitchers have a much greater bone mass in the dominant arm compared to the nondominant arm, and that dancers have more dense bones in their active legs compared to their relatively sedentary arms.

Why do amenorrheic distance runners have a lower than normal bone mineral content? Most probably, this is related to the fact that they are amenorrheic, for with the cessation of menstruation comes major alterations in reproductive hormones, hormones which are directly involved in maintaining bone health. A recent study demonstrated that amenorrheic runners did have low bone mineral contents compared to age-matched, normally menstruating, nonrunning women. However, amenorrheic nonrunners had bone mineral contents which were considerably lower. Further, runners with normal menstrual cycles had the highest levels of bone mineral content. Thus, it would appear that for optimal bone health, women should be engaged in physical activity from an early age on, in order to attain as high a bone mineral content as possible—putting bone into the bank. The hormonal changes that occur with menopause and aging lead to a gradual but consistent decrease in bone mineral. Thus, for those who stay active throughout life, there will be a larger reserve from which to draw. In addition to exercise, it may be necessary for women to increase the daily requirement for calcium to levels between 1 and 1.5 grams per day, either through the proper selection of foods or through a calcium supplement.

Exercise and Aging

Figure 19 in chapter 3 is an excellent summary of the relationship between exercise and aging. From this figure it is clear that aging is inevitable. However, equally clear is the fact that

by maintaining moderate to high levels of physical conditioning, the individual can have the physiological capacity of the
average man or woman who is 20 to 30 years younger! There
is ample evidence now that the continuation of vigorous exercise throughout life will reduce the rate of decline in the basic
physiological function of the body. What changes in body function take place as one ages?

First, the *basal metabolic rate* (BMR) decreases at a rate
of approximately 3% per decade, starting from the age of 3
through old age to death. Up to the age of 20 to 30 years, this
decreased BMR is assumed to be a reflection of a more efficient body metabolism. Beyond the age of 30 years, this
decrease is thought to reflect a decrease in the lean body tissue,
primarily muscle mass. A decrease in BMR indicates that there
will also be a decrease in the total calories that will be necessary each day to provide the energy needs of the individual.
Lung function appears to be markedly altered with age. *Pulmonary function* demonstrates a major decrease with age,
starting at between 20 and 30 years of age. The residual lung
volume increases, and the total lung capacity remains un-
changed. These changes are consistent with the reduced maximal ventilatory capacity with age in exhaustive exercise. Each
of these changes indicates a reduced efficiency and capacity
of the lungs, and is the result of a loss of elasticity of the lung
tissue and the chest wall. The decrease in mobility of the chest
wall with aging is thought to be the major cause of the reduction in lung function.

A number of changes occur in *cardiovascular function*
with aging. As was mentioned in a previous chapter, there is
a decrease in maximal heart rate with age. Cross-sectional
studies estimate the decreases to be approximately a 1-beat-
per-minute decrease each year. Recent longitudinal studies
indicate that the cross-sectional estimates may be too high.
Their data suggest a decrease of only one-half of a beat per
minute each year. Maximum stroke volume and maximum
cardiac output decrease with age, as does the capacity for
peripheral blood flow. However, it is difficult to determine how
much of this decrease is due to true aging, and how much is
the result of an increasingly sedentary life-style. Heart weight

and heart volume increase with aging, while blood volume and total hemoglobin levels tend to stay the same.

The *maximal oxygen uptake* decreases with age, as was mentioned above and illustrated in Figure 19. Peak maximal oxygen uptake values are obtained between the ages of 17 and 25 years in the male, and between 10 and 13 years in the female. The earlier onset of decline in the female is attributed to her increasingly sedentary life-style once she reaches puberty. The decrease in maximal oxygen uptake with aging is partially the result of a reduced activity level, but the reduction will occur even in those who maintain themselves in peak physical condition. This decrease which occurs irrespective of activity levels is probably the result of a reduction in maximal heart rate and cardiac output, athough the decrease in pulmonary ventilation and a decrease in maximum diffusion capacity may also be contributing factors.

Muscular strength demonstrates a linear decrease with age starting sometime between the ages of 30 and 40 years. By 60 years of age the male has not lost more than 10% to 20% of his peak maximum strength. This loss in strength is the result of inactivity as well as basic changes in the structure of muscle, which include a loss of protein due to alterations in protein synthesis.

When individuals 60 years of age and older initiate a program of exercise, the alterations in physiological function which they will experience will be similar to those experienced by individuals of a much younger age. The major difference in response to training between the younger and the older individual is in magnitude; the older individual does not respond or adapt as rapidly or to the same extent. Nonetheless, studies have shown that the individual is able to function much more efficiently in performing daily activities following a period of training.

Will vigorous exercise pursued throughout one's lifetime provide a guarantee of a longer life span? At this point in time, research data is not available to answer that question. Some have made the statement that a lifetime of vigorous exercise may not improve the quantity of life, but it certainly does improve the quality of life. While the research data is presently lacking, most scientists and clinicians who have studied this problem feel that it will only be a matter of time until evidence becomes available to indicate that the quantity of life is also increased. Until that time, most of these individuals continue their programs of vigorous activity.

C H A P T E R

Proper Nutrition for Exercise and Sport

During the 1970s nutrition became one of the most popular topics of magazine articles, books, newspaper columns, and debate. The old adage, "Never discuss or debate politics and religion," should be modified to: "Never discuss or debate politics, religion, and *nutrition*." The field of nutrition is one of extreme contrasts. On the one side are the self-proclaimed experts who have all of the answers, and on the other side are those who are truly students of nutrition who realize that the field is short on fact and long on fiction and myths. The science of nutrition has advanced considerably over the past decade, but there is still far more to be learned than is presently known. The American public is hungry for information on nutrition, and consequently, frequently falls prey to the latest fad, whether it be a new diet, a new vitamin, or a new use for an old vitamin. The gullibility of the American public in nutrition and related areas is almost beyond belief. Literally billions of dollars are spent each year as the public experiments with the latest book or gimmick on the market. In 1973, it was estimated that over $10 billion was being spent each year in the diet industry alone. Over one billion dollars was spent on special diet food. *Dr. Atkins' Diet*

Revolution sold approximately one million copies in 7 months, and Dr. Stillman's *Quick Weight Loss Diet* sold approximately five million copies in 6 years. Over $54 million was spent on "legal" diet pills alone. With the public so willing to part with its money, it is no wonder that so many charlatans have descended to grab a "piece of the action." The average consumer must be better educated and aware of the tremendous potential for fraud, misrepresentation, and misguided zeal.

The present chapter is intended to provide sound information in a highly controversial area. The major focus will be on nutrition as it relates to health, fitness, and sport. The first session will discuss the basic foundation of proper nutrition, and the second section will investigate the role of nutrition in exercise and sport. For more detailed information, a series of excellent books has been listed after the appendix under Selected Readings.

General Concepts in Nutrition

Food is composed of 6 major components: water, minerals, vitamins, proteins, fats, and carbohydrates. Each of these components is an essential ingredient in the daily diet, and has specific functions to perform to maintain the body's health equilibrium. A brief discussion of these components will allow a better understanding of the nature, importance, major sources, and recommended levels of daily intake for each.

Water

Seldom is water thought of as a food. However, it is, in many respects, the most essential of the 6 nutrients. We can go for weeks and even months without food, but we can survive without water only for a matter of a few days. Next to oxygen, it is the most important constituent for the maintenance of life. We can lose most of our fat and carbohydrate stores and half of our protein with up to a 40-pound loss of body weight and survive, but a 20% loss of body water may result in death and severe disorders occur with a loss of only 10%.

Water is a solvent in which all metabolic changes take place. It functions in digestion, absorption, circulation, and excretion. It assists in two very important regulatory functions: electrolyte balance and regulation of body temperature. In addition, water constitutes from 50% to 70% of the total body weight. Water is supplied from three major sources: fluids, foods, and metabolism. While fluid intake constitutes the major source of water (1.0 to 2.0 liters per day), a substantial amount of water is contained in food. Water constitutes 94% to 96% of lettuce, 95% of radishes, sour pickles, and celery, and 88% of an orange, as examples of a few selected foods. When food is metabolized in the body, water is an important by-product. For every 100 grams of fat, carbohydrate, or protein metabolized, the net yield of "metabolic" water is 107, 55, and 41 grams, respectively. Finally, water is eliminated from the body through the kidneys as urine, through the intestines in feces, through the skin as sweat, and through the lungs as water vapor.

Water needs will vary considerably from day to day depending on a number of factors. Two of the biggest sources of fluctuation in water needs are exercise and either, or both, high temperature and humidity. These were discussed in considerable detail in chapter 9. The major problem associated with a lack of water is dehydration, and dehydration should be avoided at all costs. It is a wise practice to consume slightly more water each day than is required by the mechanisms which control thirst. This will assure proper hydration, and any excess water will be passed off in the urine.

Minerals

Minerals have been defined nutritionally as the inorganic elements found in the body. While the body contains more than 20 minerals, approximately 17 have been proved essential in the diet. Minerals of the body are classified into two

Table 23   Mineral Elements in the Body

Mineral	Primary Location in Body	Primary Function	Food Sources
Calcium	Bones and teeth	Blood clotting, bone formation, transportation of fluids, muscle contraction	Milk and milk products, broccoli, sardines, clams, and oysters
Phosphorus	Bones and teeth	Bone formation, body's energy system, pH regulation	Cheese, egg yolk, milk, meat, fish, poultry, whole-grain cereals, legumes, and nuts
Magnesium	Bone and inside cells	Activates enzymes	Whole-grain cereals, nuts, meat, milk, green vegetables, and legumes
Sodium	Bone and extracellular fluid	Regulation of body fluid osmolarity, pH, and body fluid volume	Table salt, seafood, milk, and eggs, although abundant in most food except fruits
Chlorine	Extracellular fluid	Buffer and enzyme activation	Table salt, seafood, milk, meat, and eggs
Potassium	Intracellular fluid	Regulation of body fluid osmolarity, pH, and cell membrane transfer	Fruits, meat, milk, cereals, vegetables, and legumes
Sulfur	Amino acids	Oxidation-reduction reactions	Protein foods including meat, fish, poultry, eggs, milk, cheese, legumes, and nuts

Mineral	Function	Location in Body	Food Sources
Iron	Oxygen transportation	Hemoglobin, liver, spleen, and bone	Liver, meat, egg yolk, legumes, whole or enriched grains, dark green vegetables, shrimp, oysters
Zinc	Constituent of essential enzymes and insulin	Most tissues, with higher amounts in liver, muscle, and bone	Milk, liver, shellfish, herring, and wheat bran
Copper	Constituent of enzymes	All tissues, with larger amounts in the liver, brain, heart, and kidney	Liver, shellfish, whole grains, cherries, legumes kidney, poultry, oysters, chocolate, and nuts
Iodine	Essential constituent of thyroxin	Thyroid gland	Iodized table salt, seafood, water, and vegetables
Manganese	Constituent of essential enzymes	Bone, pituitary, liver, pancreas, and gastrointestinal tissue	Grains, nuts, legumes, fruit, and tea
Fluorine	Reduces dental caries and may reduce bone loss	Bone	Drinking water, tea, coffee, soybeans, spinach, gelatin, onions, and lettuce
Molybdenum	Constituent of essential enzymes	Enzymes	Legumes, cereal grains, dark green leafy vegetables, and organs
Cobalt	Essential to normal function of all cells	In all cells	Liver, kidney, oysters, clams, poultry, and milk
Selenium	Fat metabolism	The cell	Grains, onions, meats, milk, and vegetables
Chromium	Glucose metabolism	The cell	Corn oil, clams, whole-grain cereals, meat, and drinking water

groups: those present in relatively large amounts, and those needed in very small amounts. This latter group is referred to as the trace minerals. Those present in large amounts include sodium, potassium, calcium, phosphorus, magnesium, sulfur, and various chlorides. Of these, calcium and phosphorus in the teeth and bones account for 60% to 85% of all minerals in the body. The trace minerals include iron, zinc, selenium, manganese, iodine, copper, fluorine, and chromium.

A well-balanced diet which supplies at least 1,500 calories is typically sufficient to provide all of the body's needs for the essential minerals. With heavy exercise, several of the key minerals are lost in abundant quantities, for example, sodium chloride in sweat; however, the subsequent increase in food intake is more than sufficient to make up for these losses. Iron is the one trace mineral of which a rather sizable percentage of the population have deficiencies. Scientists have estimated that from 20% to 25% of the world's population may be deficient in iron.

Those minerals of greatest importance to body function are listed in Table 23. For each mineral listed, there is a description of the location within the body where the mineral is found, the major function of the mineral, and the best food sources for obtaining the mineral in the diet.

Vitamins

Vitamins are a group of unrelated organic compounds needed only in extremely small quantities in the diet, but essential for specific metabolic reactions within the cell, and for normal growth and maintenance of health. Vitamins were relatively unknown until the beginning of the century. Subsequently, approximately 20 vitamins have been identified, and several more have been postulated. Vitamins fall into two basic categories: those which are fat-soluble, and those which are water-soluble. Vitamins A, D, E, and K are soluble in fat, while vitamins C and B-complex vitamins are water-soluble. A fat-soluble vitamin can be stored in the liver and in the fatty tissues of the body. This is an extremely important point, for vitamin toxicity can occur when the body consumes too much

Table 24 Vitamins and Their Functions, Sources, and Associated Deficiency States

Vitamin	Primary Function	Sources	Deficiency States
FAT-SOLUBLE VITAMINS			
A	Adaptation to dim light, resistance to infection, prevents eye and skin disorders, bone and tooth development	Liver, kidney, milk, butter, egg yolk, yellow vegetables, apricots, cantaloupe, and peaches	Night blindness
D	Facilitates absorption of calcium; bone and tooth development	Sunlight, fish, eggs, fortified dairy products, and liver	Rickets
E	Prevents oxidation of essential vitamins and fatty acids and protects red blood cells from hemolysis	Wheatgerm, vegetable oils, green vegetables, milk fat, egg yolk, and nuts	No known at this time
K	Blood clotting	Liver, soybean oil, vegetable oil, green vegetables, tomatoes, cauliflower, and wheat bran	Hemorrhage disease
WATER-SOLUBLE VITAMINS			
B_1 (thiamine)	Energy metabolism, growth, appetite, and digestion	Pork, liver, organs, meat, legumes, whole-grain enriched cereals and breads, wheatgerm, and potatoes	Beriberi
B_2 (riboflavin)	Growth, health of eyes, and energy metabolism	Milk and dairy foods, organ meats, green vegetables, eggs, fish, and enriched cereals and breads	Mouth and lip lesions, loss of vision

(Cont.)

Table 24 (Cont.)

Vitamin	Primary Function	Sources	Deficiency States
Niacin	Energy metabolism and fatty acid synthesis	Fish, liver, meat, poultry, grains eggs, peanuts, milk, and legumes	Pellagra, limited energy production
B_6 (pyridoxine)	Protein metabolism and growth	Pork, glandular meats, cereal bran and germ, milk, egg yolk, oatmeal, and legumes	Convulsions, anemia
Pantothenic acid	Hemoglobin formation, and carbohydrate, protein, and fat metabolism	Whole-grain cereals, organ meats, and eggs	No known at this time
Biotin	Carbohydrate, fat, and protein metabolism	Liver, peanuts, yeast, milk, meat, egg yolk, cereal, nuts, legumes, bananas, grapefruit, tomatoes, watermelon, and strawberries	No known at this time
Folic acid (folacin)	Growth, fat metabolism, maturation of red blood cells	Green vegetables, organ meats, lean beef, wheat, eggs, fish, dry beans, lentils, asparagus, broccoli, and yeast	Anemia
B_{12} (cobalamin)	Red blood cell production, nervous system metabolism, and fat metabolism	Liver, kidney, milk and dairy foods, and meat	Anemia, neuro-muscular weakness
C (ascorbic acid)	Growth, tissue repair, tooth and bone formation	Citrus fruits, tomatoes, strawberries, potatoes, melons, peppers, and pineapple	Scurvy

of a specific fat-soluble vitamin over long periods of time. Vitamins A and D have been shown to be the most common of the fat-soluble vitamins to exhibit significant impairment of bodily function with toxicity. Water-soluble vitamins are soluble in water, and, as such, they cannot be stored in the body, and any excessive intake of these vitamins will only find their way into the urine and out of the body. With an annual consumption of $300 million to $500 million worth of vitamin supplements each year, our country must produce the most expensive urine in the world. Most, if not all, vitamin supplementation is unnecessary. This will be discussed later. The vitamins, their sources and functions, and the problems associated with deficiencies are listed in Table 24.

Proteins

Protein was the first substance recognized as a vital part of living tissue, and is now known to be the fundamental structural compound of cells, antibodies, enzymes, and many hormones. Most protein is located in muscle tissue, but it is also distributed in the soft tissues, bone, teeth, blood, and other body fluids. Proteins are comprised of at least 23 different amino acids, of which between 8 and 10 are referred to as essential amino acids. The essential amino acids are those which can't be synthesized by the body, and are therefore essential to include in the diet. If there is a shortage or deficiency of any of these essential amino acids, there will be serious limitations placed on growth and general body function. Proteins are derived from both animal tissue and from the seeds, or grains, of plants. Those who are on vegetarian, or modified vegetarian, diets will be able to obtain the essential amino acids providing their food choices are selected carefully. A lacto-vegetarian diet (includes milk and milk products) or a lacto-ovo-vegetarian diet (includes eggs as well as milk and milk products) provides an even greater opportunity for meeting the basic requirements for protein as well as the other essential nutrients.

Proteins serve many critical functions in the body. They are used in repairing tissue which has become worn out from constant use, as well as in building new tissue. The amino acids are considered to be the building blocks of tissue, and protein is their only source. Proteins are involved in almost all body secretions and fluids, including enzymes, some hormones, mucus, milk, and sperm. Proteins also are important in the body's osmotic reactions which control fluid volumes, in the body's resistance to disease through antibodies, and in the body's blood-clotting mechanism. Finally, hemoglobin, which is the oxygen carrier in the blood, is composed of iron (heme) and a large protein molecule (globin).

Approximately 5% to 15% of the total calories ingested per day are from protein. It has been estimated that the average American consumes between two and three times the total amount of protein that is needed. This excess is totally unnecessary, expensive, and is potentially harmful. The daily recommended allowances published in 1980 by the National Research Council for the average man and woman are 56 and 44 grams of protein per day, respectively, which are reduced from the 1968 recommendations of 65 and 55 grams per day. These recommendations are for the average-sized person, a 70-kilogram (154 -pound) man and a 55-kilogram (120-pound) woman. The recommended intake would be increased or decreased proportionally depending on body weight. For the mature adult, an allowance of approximately 0.8 grams per kilogram of body weight is considered appropriate.

Fats

Fats or lipids are terms used to define a similar group of compounds which are insoluble in water, soluble in organic solvents such as ether and chloroform, and utilizable by living organisms. A fat consists of two different clusters of atoms: *glycerol* and *fatty acid*. When glycerol and fatty acid molecules are bound chemically, they form triglycerides. Most natural fats are composed of between 98% and 99% triglyceride. Lipids are generally classified into one of three categories:

simple, compound, and derived. Simple lipids include fatty acids, neutral fats (including triglycerides), and waxes. Compound lipids include phospholipids, glycolipids, and lipoproteins. Derived lipids include mono- and di-glycerides, glycerol, sterols (including cholesterol), and fat-soluble vitamins. Chapters 1 and 2 included a detailed discussion of cholesterol and its relationship to coronary artery disease, with specific reference to the lipoprotein carriers of cholesterol.

There are two types of fatty acids: *saturated* and *unsaturated*. The difference between the two is in the bonding between carbon and hydrogen atoms. Unsaturated fats contain one (monounsaturated) or more (polyunsaturated) double bonds between carbon atoms in a chain of carbon atoms. Each double bond in the chain takes the place of two hydrogen atoms. When the carbon chain is saturated with hydrogen atoms— two hydrogen atoms for each carbon atom—this is referred to as a saturated fatty acid. In practical terms, a saturated fat is in the form of a solid such as animal fat, and an unsaturated fat is in the form of a liquid, such as fish and vegetable oil. By the process of hydrogenation, unsaturated oils can be changed from a liquid to a semi-solid state. Saturated fats are derived primarily from animal sources, including the fat in meats such as beef, lamb, pork, and chicken, and in egg and dairy products such as egg yolk, milk, cream, and cheese. Unsaturated fats are derived primarily from plant sources.

Fat is an extremely important energy source both at rest and during light to moderate exercise. Fats are the most concentrated source of food energy in the diet, providing over twice the number of calories per unit of weight than either carbohydrates or proteins. Fat is also easily stored, and is a ready source of energy under almost all conditions. Fat is the only source of linoleic acid, and is the mode of transportation in the body for the fat-soluble vitamins. Fat plays an important part in the regulation of body temperature, since it is an excellent insulator. While this works to the advantage of the individual in cold weather, it is a distinct disadvantage during the hot weather months. Fat also serves to protect the vital organs such as the heart, liver, kidneys, spleen, brain, and spinal cord. Finally, fat adds palatability to food, and due to its slow passage from the stomach it tends to satiate the appetite, or reduce the feeling of hunger, for long periods of time.

Fat constitutes approximately 45% of the total calories consumed in the diet of the average American today, which is a considerably higher percentage of fat intake compared to that at the turn of this century. Current recommendations suggest that fat should constitute only 25% to 30% of our total calories, and that the reductions in fat intake should come from saturated fats. There is presently a great deal of controversy on specific recommendations for the intake of saturated fats, particularly in reference to egg and dairy products as they relate to coronary artery disease.

Carbohydrates

Carbohydrates are represented by the various sugars and starches, and are the most efficient, and usually the least expensive, source of food energy. They are classified as monosaccharides, disaccharides, and polysaccharides. Glucose, fructose, galactose, and mannose are the monosaccharides, or simple sugars. Disaccharides are double sugars, or the bonding of two simple monosaccharides, and are exemplified by sucrose (glucose plus fructose), maltose (glucose plus glucose), and lactose (glucose plus galactose). Sucrose is ordinary table sugar and is found mainly in sugar cane and sugar beets. Polysaccharides are composed of three or more monosaccharides and include starch and glycogen. Glycogen is the form in which glucose is stored in the body. The term *glycogenesis* refers to the process of transforming glucose to glycogen, while *glycogenolysis* refers to the breakdown of glycogen to glucose in the liver.

In addition to being a ready energy source, and a particularly important fuel source for high-intensity exercise, carbohydrates also exert an influence on both protein and fat metabolism, sparing the use of protein as an energy source, and controlling the amount of fat that is utilized. Glucose is critical as the sole energy source for the brain and is essential for maintenance of the functional integrity of the nervous system.

Carbohydrates constitute approximately 50% to 60% of the total dietary calories consumed by the average American, but this percentage has been decreasing since the early 1900s. This reduction has come from a decreased intake of starches, for the intake of sugars has actually increased. The major sources of sugars and starches are grains, fruits, vegetables, milk, and concentrated sweets. Refined sugar, syrup, and cornstarch are examples of pure carbohydrates, and many of the concentrated sweets such as candy, honey, jellies, molasses, and soft drinks contain few, if any, other nutrients. These have been referred to as "empty calories" since they contribute nothing but calories to the diet.

Recommended Dietary Allowances

In the 1940s, the potential for nutrition-related health problems was recognized and the Food and Nutrition Board of the National Research Council of the National Academy of Sciences was formed and published the first report known as the *Recommended Dietary Allowances*, or RDA. These original recommendations are revised periodically, and they are intended to provide guidelines for planning and evaluating food intake. These recommended allowances are specified for total energy intake, and for protein, vitamin, and mineral intake. The recommendations are based on the age and sex of the individual, and include the special circumstances of pregnant and lactating women. The 1980 RDA's are provided in Table 25. With the new practice of labeling the nutrient contents of most packaged foods, these RDA's have much more meaning and significance. Still, the numbers and unfamiliar units of measure make these recommendations of limited value for most individuals, and eventually led the Department of Agriculture to create and publish a simplified plan, titled "The Essentials of an Adequate Diet."

This publication provided a much more simplified approach to diet and menu planning. The "Four-Food-Group Plan" establishes recommendations for daily food intake in each of four basic areas: milk and milk products; meat and

Table 25   Recommended Daily Dietary Allowances,[a] 1980.[b]

Designed for the maintenance of good nutrition of practically all healthy people in the U.S.A.

	Age	Weight		Height		Energy	Protein	Vit. A Activity	Fat-Soluble Vitamins			
									Vit. A	Vit. D	Vit. E Activity[f]	Vit. K
	(years)	(kg)	(lbs)	(cm)	(in)	(kcal)[c]	(g)	(µg RE)[d]	(IU)	(IU)	(IU)	(µg)
Infants	0.0-0.5	6	13	60	24	kg×115	kg×2.2	420[e]	1,400	400	3	12
	0.5-1.0	9	20	71	28	kg×105	kg×2.0	400	2,000	400	4	10-20
Children	1-3	13	29	90	35	1,300	23	400	2,000	400	5	15-30
	4-6	20	44	112	44	1,700	30	500	2,500	400	6	20-40
	7-10	28	62	132	52	2,400	34	700	3,300	400	7	30-60
Males	11-14	45	99	157	62	2,700	45	1,000	5,000	400	8	50-100
	15-18	66	145	176	70	2,800	56	1,000	5,000	400	10	50-100
	19-22	70	154	177	70	2,900	56	1,000	5,000	300	10	70-140
	23-50	70	154	178	70	2,700	56	1,000	5,000	200	10	70-140
	51+	70	154	178	70	2,400	56	1,000	5,000	200	10	70-140
Females	11-14	46	101	157	62	2,200	46	800	4,000	400	8	50-100
	15-18	55	120	163	64	2,100	46	800	4,000	400	8	50-100
	19-22	55	120	163	64	2,100	44	800	4,000	400	8	70-140
	23-50	55	120	163	64	2,000	44	800	4,000	200	8	70-140
	51+	55	120	163	64	1,800	44	800	4,000	200	8	70-140
Pregnant						+300	+30	+200	+1,000	+200	+2	
Lactating						+500	+20	+400	+2,000	+200	+3	

[a] The allowances are intended to provide for individual variations among most normal persons as they live in the United States under usual environmental stresses. Diets should be based on a variety of common foods in order to provide other nutrients for which human requirements have been less well defined.

[b] From the Food and Nutrition Board, National Research Council of the National Academy of Sciences.

[c] Kilojoules (kJ)—4.2 × kcal.

[d] Retinol equivalents.

(Cont.)

Table 25 (Cont.)

| Age (years) | Water-Soluble Vitamins | | | | | | | | | Minerals | | | |
	Ascorbic Acid (mg)	Folacin[c] (µg)	Niacin (mg)	Riboflavin (mg)	Thiamin (mg)	Vit. B₆ (mg)	Vit. B₁₂ (µg)	Calcium (mg)	Phosphorus (mg)	Iodine (µg)	Iron (mg)	Magnesium (mg)	Zinc (mg)
Infants													
0.0-0.5	35	30	6	0.4	0.3	0.3	0.5	360	240	40	10	50	3
0.5-1.0	35	45	8	0.6	0.5	0.6	1.5	540	360	50	15	70	5
Children													
1-3	45	100	9	0.8	0.7	0.9	2.0	800	800	70	15	150	10
4-6	45	200	11	1.0	0.9	1.3	2.5	800	800	90	10	200	10
7-10	45	300	16	1.4	1.2	1.6	3.0	800	800	120	10	250	10
Males													
11-14	50	400	18	1.6	1.4	1.8	3.0	1,200	1,200	150	18	350	15
15-18	60	400	18	1.7	1.4	2.0	3.0	1,200	1,200	150	18	400	15
19-22	60	400	19	1.7	1.5	2.2	3.0	800	800	150	10	350	15
23-50	60	400	18	1.6	1.4	2.2	3.0	800	800	150	10	350	15
51+	60	400	16	1.4	1.2	2.2	3.0	800	800	150	10	350	15
Females													
11-14	50	400	15	1.3	1.1	1.8	3.0	1,200	1,200	150	18	300	15
15-18	60	400	14	1.3	1.1	2.0	3.0	1,200	1,200	150	18	300	15
19-22	60	400	14	1.3	1.1	2.0	3.0	800	800	150	18	300	15
23-50	60	400	13	1.2	1.0	2.0	3.0	800	800	150	18	300	15
51+	60	400	13	1.2	1.0	2.0	3.0	800	800	150	10	300	15
Pregnant	+20	+400	+2	+0.3	+0.4	+0.6	+1.0	+400	+400	+25	30	+150	+5
Lactating	+40	+100	+5	+0.5	+0.5	+0.5	+1.0	+400	+400	+50	+30	+150	+10

[a] Assumed to be all as retinol in milk during the first six months of life. All subsequent intakes are assumed to be half as retinol and half as β-carotene when calculated from international units. As retinol equivalents, three fourths are as retinol and one fourth as β-carotene.

[b] Total vitamin E activity estimated to be 80 percent as α-tocopherol and 20 percent other tocopherols.

[c] The folacin allowances refer to dietary sources as determined by *Lactobacillus casei* assay. Pure forms of folacin may be effective in doses less than one fourth of the recommended dietary allowance.

high-protein foods; fruits and vegetables; and cereals and grain foods. Table 26 outlines the "Four-Food-Group Plan," including the number of servings per day and the major contributions of each food group. It should be emphasized that these recommendations are based on meeting the minimal requirements, and will have to be increased either by larger or more servings for individuals who are active and expend a considerable amount of additional energy each day. The individual with a weight problem, however, should take a close look at Table 25 to determine if the total number of calories taken in each day exceeds the RDA for sex, weight, and age. If a reduction in calories is recommended, this should be accomplished by reducing the size of the servings in all food groups and not by reducing the number of servings in any one group.

Table 26 The Basic "Four-Food-Group Plan"

Food Group	Daily Amounts for Adults	Nutritional Contribution
Milk and Milk Products	Two or more servings per day either as a milk beverage or a milk product such as cheese and ice cream; a serving would be one cup or its equivalent	Protein Calcium Riboflavin Vitamin D
Meat and High-Protein Products	Two or more servings of meat, fish, poultry, eggs, or vegetables such as dried beans, lentils, peas, and nuts; a serving of meat, fish, or poultry would be 3.5 ounces of lean and boneless meat	Protein Thiamin Iron Niacin Riboflavin
Fruits and Vegetables	Four or more servings per day of ½ cup or more	Vitamin A Vitamin C Folic acid
Cereals and Grains	Four or more servings per day with one serving equal to one slice of bread, ½ to ¾ cup of cooked cereal, macaroni, spaghetti, etc.	Protein Thiamin Riboflavin Niacin Iron

A balanced diet is the goal or objective for the total population, and should include approximately 10% to 15% protein, 30% to 35% fat, and 50% to 60% carbohydrate, minimizing saturated fat and concentrated sugars.

Dietary Supplements

The food industry makes a considerable amount of money each year in the area of dietary supplements. Is there a need for vitamin and mineral supplementation? What advantages are to be gained from protein supplementation? It would appear that for the individual who is getting a well-balanced diet, and is moderately active, dietary supplementation is totally unnecessary. This is a highly controversial area, for literally thousands of people can give personal testimonies as to how much help they received and how much better they feel from supplementing one or more of the vitamins. It is difficult, if not impossible, to refute these claims. However, the basic research which is highly controlled to avoid personal biases would indicate that such claims are unfounded. This is not to deny that some good may have been achieved in some individuals, but the research literature overwhelmingly supports the position that supplements are not necessary. Logically, supplements would not be expected to provide any benefits. With the exception of the fat-soluble vitamins, supplementation of water-soluble vitamins and minerals will not result in any long-term effects since they are rapidly excreted in the urine. Protein is already being consumed in the diet at levels in excess of two to three times that which is needed. Further supplementation of protein will have no additional benefits.

What about the athlete or recreational jogger? Won't their needs for additional vitamins, minerals, and protein be increased as they increase their total caloric expenditure above that of the moderately active individual? In reality, the answer to this question is no. The protein requirement will go up in proportion to the additional energy that is being expended each day, but the increased food intake will more than take care of the increased requirement. The recommendations for most vitamins and minerals are established independent of exercise habits; increased levels of activity essentially don't alter the basic requirements. In addition, the food intake tends to parallel the level of activity, so the individual who exercises vigorously each day is probably taking in far more vitamins than needed. Supplementation may be necessary, however, for the individual who is on a calorie-restricted diet. When the total calorie intake per day decreases to 1,500 calories or less, there may be need for a general multi-vitamin.

Nutrition in Exercise and Sport

For centuries man has related his success or failure in athletics to what he ate or drank either before or during competition. Mystical qualities have been ascribed to buffalo meat, dessicated liver, bee pollen, fructose, amino acid supplements, honey, and numerous other foods, vitamins, or minerals. Is it possible to manipulate the diet to achieve an improvement in performance? The answer to that question is a qualified yes, although improvement is limited to the manipulation in only one or two nutritional areas, and the degree of improvement is still debatable. Unfortunately, so much of the research that has been conducted in this area has lacked adequate controls. It is appropriate to use the double-blind technique for this type of research, where neither the subject in the study nor the principle scientist or investigator has knowledge as to which group is receiving a certain dietary supplement and which is receiving a placebo. Only after the study has been completed does a third party come forward with the key as to who received what treatment. While this is the most appropriate technique to use, few studies have employed it, which leaves one highly suspicious of those studies which failed to use this technique.

Protein Supplements

As was discussed in detail in the previous section, the average diet in America today contains two to three times more protein than is required on a daily basis. Since the amino acids of protein are the essential building blocks for the growth and development of body tissue, it has been the tradition over the years to liberally supplement protein when attempting to achieve increase in muscle bulk and strength through intensive strength training programs. Will this additional supplementation, over and above the excess protein in the normal diet, substantially increase muscle bulk? Logic, and most nutritionists, would answer an emphatic no! However, several recent studies indicate the protein supplementation may increase body protein stores and muscle mass. In one study, two groups of young men were engaged in heavy physical activity, consuming either 1.4 or 2.8 grams of protein per day for every kilogram of body weight for a period of 40 days. The group receiving the increased level of protein did have substantially greater gains in muscle mass and body protein storage. Studies investigating the influence of anabolic steroids in promoting gains in muscular strength and size found that the steroids were ineffective unless they were accompanied by a protein supplement. It would appear that protein supplementation may facilitate the growth of muscle, although the gains are not considerable, and probably do not justify the tremendous expense associated with the commercial supplements.

Fat and Carbohydrate

While at one time carbohydrate was considered the primary, if not the only, fuel for muscular exercise, it is now recognized that the role of fat as a primary energy source during exercise is considerable. Fat is essentially an inexhaustible source of fuel, while carbohydrate stores are greatly limited, providing for not more than 60 to 120 minutes of moderately heavy exercise. Since the stores of carbohydrate are limited, it would facilitate performance if either or both carbohydrate stores could be increased, or if fat could be utilized in place of carbohydrate, sparing carbohydrate stores, and theoretically prolonging endurance exercise.

With this in mind, Scandinavian researchers in the 1960s experimented with various combinations of diet and endurance performance. In one study, the subjects were placed on a specific dietary regimen for 3-day intervals and tested on an all-out ride to exhaustion on a cycle ergometer at a work load that represented 75% of the individual's capacity, or maximal oxygen uptake. The total work time on the ergometer was directly related to the glycogen content in the exercising muscles, and the glycogen content varied in direct response to the diet. After a normal mixed diet, the subjects worked for nearly 126 minutes before they reached exhaustion, and the initial glycogen content in the exercising muscles was 1.93 grams per 100 grams of wet tissue. After 3 days on a diet of fat and protein, with very limited carbohydrate, the subjects' initial glycogen content was 0.69 grams per 100 grams of wet tissue, and the riding time to exhaustion was reduced to only 59 minutes. After an additional 3 days on a high-carbohydrate diet, the subjects started the ride with a glycogen content of 3.70 grams per 100 grams of wet tissue, and were able to prolong the time to exhaustion for the same intensity of exercise to 189 minutes, an improvement of approximately 50% above that for the normal diet, and more than a threefold increase over the high-fat and high-protein diet.

These findings were not totally unexpected, however, since earlier work had shown that exhaustion from endurance exercise was accompanied by hypoglycemia, or low blood sugar, and by low, if not totally depleted, glycogen stores in the active muscles. Subsequent studies have verified this rather remarkable response to nutritional manipulation. In one study, subjects participated in two 30-kilometer cross-country running races, one after a normal mixed diet, and the other following several days on an extremely high-carbohydrate diet. The high-carbohydrate diet resulted in initial muscle glycogen levels that were nearly double the levels attained following the mixed diet, and in substantially improved race times, with the improvement coming essentially in the last half of the race.

This elevation of glycogen stores through nutritional manipulation has been referred to as carbohydrate loading. Subsequent research and self-experimentation by athletes themselves have refined the carbohydrate loading technique. The athlete must totally deplete carbohydrate stores approximately 7 to 8 days prior to the day of competition by a high-intensity workout of 60 to 120 minutes in duration. This is then followed by 3 to 4 days of reduced activity and a very low-carbohydrate diet. The final 3 to 4 days prior to competition is the time during which the carbohydrate stores are replenished with a very high-carbohydrate diet, and little or no activity. These last few days are the athlete's reward for all the hard training and that very difficult period of restriction to a very low-carbohydrate intake. Some athletes omit the period of low-carbohydrate intake. This is a much easier regimen to follow, and probably doesn't reduce the overall benefits that much. Recent studies suggest that neither the all-out bout of exercise or the period of low carbohydrate intake are necessary to achieve the optimal effect. Simply tapering the intensity and duration of the training program to low levels the last 5 to 7 days prior to competition, coupled with a high carbohydrate diet the final 3 to 4 days, appears to provide the same benefits. Angina-like symptoms (chest pain) have been noted in several athletes who have attempted carbohydrate loading. It is unclear as to whether this was truly a cardiovascular problem, or, if it was a cardiovascular problem, whether it was related to carbohydrate loading. Recognizing the potential for problems, athletes who attempt this nutritional manipulation should proceed with caution.

The second method in which endurance performance might be facilitated is by shifting the primary energy source from carbohydrate to fat, thus sparing the limited carbohydrate for use later in the exercise. At rest and during exercise, the energy source is seldom from a single fuel, but, rather, is a combination of both fat and carbohydrate. As the intensity of exercise shifts from low or moderate levels to high or exhaustive levels, a greater fraction of the energy is derived from carbohydrate. At any given intensity, if the body could be manipulated to use a higher fraction of fat as the energy source, carbohydrates would be spared, and the individual should, theoretically, be able to prolong the length of the exercise period prior to reaching the state of exhaustion. This theory was tested on both animals and humans, and it was found that increasing the levels of free fatty acids in the blood by either heparin or caffeine increased the utilization of fats and spared the limited carbohydrate stores, thereby increasing the capacity for prolonged endurance exercise. The amount of caffeine needed to accomplish the effect is approximately the equivalent of two cups of coffee, ingested 30 to 60 minutes prior to exercise.

Vitamins and Minerals

Numerous research studies have been conducted to determine the benefits, if any, from the supplementation of various vitamins and minerals. There are a number of studies which indicate some improvement in performance with specific vitamin supplementation, but there are nearly an equal number of studies which show essentially no benefits. In reviewing all of these studies, it would appear that several of the B-complex vitamins, and vitamins C and E, may provide limited beneficial effects if supplemented, but this conclusion is certainly open to debate. If there is improvement from supplementation of these vitamins, the magnitude of improvement would be very small.

The supplementation of minerals, particularly salt in the form of salt tablets, has been advocated for a number of years. With the loss of salt in sweat, it was theorized that supplementation of salt through salt tablets was essential. It is now recognized that the average individual gets sufficient salt in his or her diet, even in hot and humid weather when the volume of sweat lost per day is increased considerably. One of the basic adaptations the body makes to heat stress is to reduce the salt content of the sweat, thereby conserving salt. A liberal salting of food is now considered to be sufficient for replacing that salt which was lost. Salt tablets are not advocated, for they could promote the retention of water and the loss of potassium, in addition to having potentially dangerous side effects for persons with high blood pressure. Aspartates, which are potassium and magnesium salts of aspartic acid, have been promoted as a beneficial supplement on the basis of their interaction with blood ammonia. Again, studies are nearly evenly divided as to whether supplementation has any value in improving athletic performance.

Pre-Contest Meal

It has been traditional for the athlete to have a thick, juicy steak, baked potato, and salad as the pre-contest meal. It is now recognized that this is probably the worst possible meal the athlete could eat prior to competition. Steak has a relatively high fat content, and fat slows down the total digestive process. With food still in the stomach and intestine during exercise, this sets up a competition for the available blood supply between the gastrointestinal area and the muscles that are involved in competition. Also the pre-competition tension or anxiety also tends to slow the digestive process, and a heavy meal will frequently lead to nausea and vomiting. As a result, more athletes are switching to very light meals 3 to 4 hours prior to competition, and saving their steak for either the night before or the night after competition. Those who practice carbohydrate loading typically have an extremely large dinner the evening before a race. Traditionally, this has included plates of spaghetti, loaves of bread, and much beer and wine. Since most long-distance races are conducted early in the morning to escape the heat of the day, the large meal the night before competition is probably not advisable. It typically leaves the runner feeling very full and uncomfortable, with the need for a large bowel movement, which hopefully can be accomplished prior to the start of the race. This large meal is traditional and enjoyable, but should be moved back 6 to 24 hours, either to the preceding dinner or lunch, respectively.

The use of a liquid pre-contest meal is becoming popular. A liquid diet is palatable, digests relatively easily, leaves the stomach and intestine quickly, provides the essential nutrients, and is less likely to result in nervous indigestion, nausea, vomiting, and abdominal cramps. This would appear to be a wise choice for a pre-contest meal on the basis of that information presently available. However, each athlete has his or her own personal preferences and beliefs, and to disturb these may have a much greater negative influence than the positive influence of the liquid diet.

For those athletes who are participating in endurance contests which last for several hours or more, there is probably a need to supplement glucose in the fluids they consume for water and electrolyte replacement. After several hours of endurance exercise, the blood sugar level starts to fall. This can be prevented by the addition of small quantities of glucose to the fluid replacement solution, not to exceed 2.5 grams per 100 milliliters of solution. Glucose in excess of this concentration begins to limit the rate at which the solution empties from the stomach. This reduces the rate of fluid replacement, which is highly undesirable, since fluid replacement is the primary concern relative to the health and safety of the athlete.

12

C H A P T E R

Prevention and Treatment of Athletic Injuries

The competitive athlete, the recreational athlete, and the individual who is exercising to achieve health-related benefits all have something in common. At one time or another, each will experience an athletic, sport, or exercise-related injury. This may be an injury as serious as a skull fracture or direct blow to the kidney, or it may be something as minor as a simple ankle sprain or a blister on the bottom of the foot. Injuries are, at the least, an inconvenience and a distraction from optimal performance, but they can be devastating, ending in permanent disability or death. Like many diseases, most athletic injuries are preventable, providing the proper precautions are taken in advance. This chapter will discuss the various types of injuries that occur as a result of exercise and sport, list the most common medical problems associated with specific sports, present the most appropriate steps for preventing injury, and, finally, discuss the appropriate techniques for the acute treatment of injuries. Since the area of athletic injuries is so vast in scope, this chapter will, by necessity, be limited to a summary of the major points.

Types of Athletic Injuries

Dr. Thomas Fahey, in his book *What to Do About Athletic Injuries*, states that there are four basic types of athletic injuries: sudden traumatic injuries; repeated traumatic injuries; overuse injuries; and imbalance injuries. A quick blow to the side of the head or a fracture of the femur would be classified as sudden traumatic injuries. A knee which is wrenched in one play in the football game and continuously subjected to trauma on subsequent plays until the player finally has to remove himself from the game is an example of a repeated trauma injury. Overuse injuries are injuries which result from repetitive movements where the individual isn't properly trained for that level of stress, or where improper techniques are used. Tennis elbow and jogger's knee are examples of overuse injuries. Imbalance injuries are the result of postural imbalances, anatomical weaknesses, and overdevelopment of certain muscle groups at the expense of others.

Exposed and Unexposed Wounds

Most injuries fall into one of two categories: exposed wounds, and unexposed wounds. Exposed wounds include abrasions, lacerations, incisions, and puncture wounds. *Abrasions* are those conditions where the skin is abraded or scraped against a rough surface. The outer layers of skin are torn away, exposing numerous capillaries. *Lacerations* are the result of a sharp or pointed object tearing the tissue, giving the wound an appearance of a jagged-edged cavity. *Puncture wounds* involve the direct penetration of the skin and underlying tissues by a sharp-pointed object, such as a spike or cleat on an athletic shoe. *Incisions* are clean cuts which are frequently the result of a direct blow over a sharp or poorly padded bone.

Unexposed wounds, or closed wounds, are those internal injuries in which the outer layer of skin hasn't been penetrated. These wounds include contusions, strains, sprains, dislocations, and fractures. *Contusions* are bruises, and are the result of traumatic blows to the body. Contusions can be relatively minor or superficial in nature, or they can be major, involving deep tissue tears and hemorrhage. The discoloration which appears within 24 to 48 hours is the result of the hemorrhage which forms a hematoma, or blood clot. Most contusions are relatively minor, and if treated immediately will present few, if any, problems other than localized soreness. Major contusions, however, are much more painful and require considerable time to heal. Football players receive contusions of the thigh as a result of a sharp block or tackle. These are typically tender and extremely painful if direct contact is made with them before they have fully healed.

Strains are commonly referred to as muscle pulls, and represent a tear or rip in the muscle itself or the adjacent tissue. Strains may result from simple minute separations of connective tissue and muscle fiber, to a complete avulsion or pulling away of the tendon from its bony attachment. Strains are most common in the hamstrings group, gastrocnemius, quadriceps group, hip flexors, hip adductor group, the spinalis group of the back, the deltoid, and the rotator cuff group of the shoulder. A snapping sound may be heard when the tissue tears, which is followed immediately by a sharp pain, and loss of function and severe weakness result. Frequently, spasmodic contractions occur, the specific injured area is very tender to the touch, and an indentation or cavity can be felt where the tissues have separated.

Sprains are the result of a traumatic twisting of the joint which results in either a stretching or tearing of the stabilizing connective tissues, and represent one of the most common, and frequently one of the most disabling, athletic injuries. In some cases, a severe sprain is much more disabling and takes longer to heal than a fracture in the same general area. With sprains, there is injury to the surrounding ligaments, to the articular capsule and synovial membrane, and to the tendons crossing the joint. Blood and synovial fluid leak into the joint cavity, causing swelling, extreme tenderness, and a limited range of motion. The joints which are most vulnerable to sprain include the ankles, knees, shoulders, wrists, fingers, and elbows.

Dislocations result when the joint is forced to go beyond its normal anatomical limitations. Subluxations are partial dislocations in which the separation between two articulating bones is incomplete. Luxations are complete dislocations, in which there is complete separation between two articulating bones. With dislocations, there is an immediate loss of limb function, deformity of the joint is almost always apparent, and swelling and tenderness are immediately present.

Fractures are defined as interruptions in the continuity of the bone, and are classified as either simple or compound. A simple fracture involves a break in the bone without breaking through the skin, whereas in a compound fracture, the bone extends through the outer layers of the skin, which then is classified as an external wound. Fractures can be further classified into these additional categories. *Comminuted fractures* consist of three or more bone fragments at the fracture site. *Depressed fractures* occur in flat bones such as those comprising the skull. *Greenstick fractures* are incomplete breaks in bones that have not yet completed ossification. *Impacted fractures* are those in which long bones telescope one part of the bone on another, resulting from tremendous forces applied through the long axis of the bone. *Longitudinal fractures* are those in which the bone splits along its length. *Multiple fractures* involve a severe break and separation of bone sections. *Oblique fractures* are breaks which occur at an oblique angle to the long axis of the bone. *Serrated fractures* are those in which there are two bony fragments, each having a sawtoothed, sharp-edged fracture line. *Spiral fractures* give the appearance of a spiral, or S-shaped, separation. *Transverse fractures* occur in a straight line, at right angles to the long axis of the bone. *Stress fractures* are hairline breaks in bone which are the result of overuse or sudden trauma. Stress fractures are sometimes missed on the initial diagnosis, only to show up on later X rays. When a stress fracture is suspected, an X ray should be taken several weeks following the initial complaint.

Other Injuries

Several other injuries or problems which do not fall under the classification of wounds include muscle soreness, muscle cramps, muscle spasms, tendinitis, bursitis, blisters, bone bruises, shin splints, and chondromalacia patella. *Muscle soreness* was discussed in chapter 7, and it was mentioned that the specific cause of muscle soreness is still to be determined. Soreness almost always is involved when a muscle or muscle group is exercised above the intensity at which it is normally exercised, and usually is associated with eccentric muscle contractions, when the muscle is lengthening. *Muscle cramps* may be due to a salt, potassium and or calcium ion imbalance in the muscle. *Muscle spasm* is a term used synonymously with muscle cramps. *Tendinitis* is an inflammation of the sheath which covers the tendon, and is frequently the result of overuse. *Bursitis* refers to inflammation of the bursa, which are closed sacs that contain fluid, and are strategically located in areas of the body where friction or shock occur, such as between a tendon and the underlying bone. *Blisters* are usually the result of excessive friction between the skin and some external surface, such as a shoe. The epidermis separates from the dermis and fluid accumulates between the two layers of skin. *Bone bruises* are painful contusions of bone, most typically the bones of the feet. *Shin splints* refer to a sharp pain along the front aspect of the shin bone or tibia, and are probably the result of a lowered arch, irritated membranes, separation of the muscle from the bone, hairline fracture of the bone, or other factors. *Chondromalacia patella* is a very painful, disabling knee injury which is the result of continued irritation and a breaking down of the undersurface of the patella or kneecap. This is a very common complaint among distance runners, and can be traced, in many cases, to running on a sloped surface where the kneecap is forced to take an unnatural path as it moves through the range of motion.

Medical Problems Associated With Specific Sports

In a recent book, Dr. John Bergfeld, team physician for the Cleveland Browns professional football team and orthopedic surgeon at the prestigious Cleveland Clinic, listed all of the common medical problems faced by athletes in various sports, due to trauma, overuse, environmental factors, and illness. Figures 27 and 28 illustrate where on the body these specific injuries occur.

Prevention of Athletic Injuries

One of the first steps in preventing injury is to be familiar with the major types of injuries which characterize a specific sport or activity. Recognizing the potential for injury alerts all of us to be particularly sensitive to and avoid, if possible, those factors which might lead to such an injury. Ankle sprains are one of the more common medical problems in basketball. Recognizing this, many basketball teams require their athletes to tape their ankles in an attempt to provide greater stability to the joint, and to reduce the risk of serious ankle sprains. This is referred to as *preventive taping*.

The *equipment* that is used in the specific activity must be properly fitted and wisely selected. A major problem exists in the sport of football relative to the design and construction of helmets. Individual lawsuits for hundreds of thousands, and even millions, of dollars have been filed against equipment manufacturers for the faulty design of the protective headwear, which resulted in serious injury, and even death. The design and construction of the helmet may not have been the problem at all. It may have simply been a matter of a poor fit, or the alignment of the body at the time of impact. A poorly fitting shoe will cause the jogger continual problems of an annoying, and possibly incapacitating, nature—problems which could have been avoided with a proper fitting.

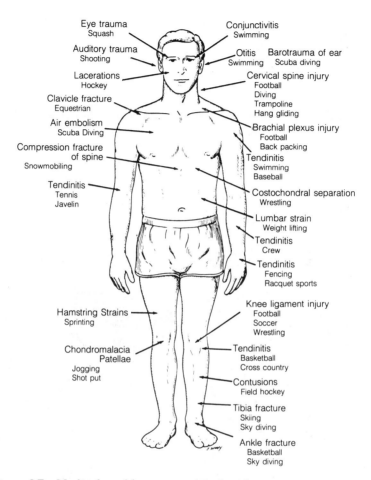

Figure 27 Medical problems associated with various sports[1]

---

[1]Reproduced with permission from Wilmore, J.H., & Bergfeld, J. (1979). A comparison of sports: Physiological and medical aspects. In Strauss, R.H. (Ed.), *Sports medicine and physiology*. Philadelphia: W.B. Saunders.

Figure 28   Medical problems associated with various sports[1]

[1]Reproduced with permission from Wilmore, J.H., & Bergfeld, J. (1979). A comparison of sports: Physiological and medical aspects. In Strauss, R.H. (Ed.), *Sports medicine and physiology*. Philadelphia: W.B. Saunders.

The *environment* is also a major factor associated with injuries, and can be controlled to a certain extent. The playing surface is responsible for many injuries. Holes or ruts on fields, sand on bicycle paths, and water on the basketball or tennis court are just a few of many examples of how the playing surface can contribute to the injury. A careful survey of the existing conditions prior to getting swept up in the enthusiasm of the competition can prevent serious injury. The weather conditions are also an extemely important factor which can significantly contribute to the increased risk of injury. As was discussed in chapter 9, there are serious heat- and cold-related injuries which can be prevented by proper hydration, appropriate clothing, the scheduling of workouts or competition at a time of day when the weather conditions will be more favorable, and even canceling or postponing a workout or competition if the weather conditions exceed a certain critical level. The time of day one exercises or competes is also associated with increased or decreased risk for injury. Exercise should be avoided in the heat of the day, or at that time of day when pollution levels are at their peak. Jogging or bicycling on city streets during rush-hour traffic should also be avoided. Finally, if exercise is performed at a time when it is dark, either in the evening or early morning, precautions should be taken to assure proper lighting to avoid tripping or stumbling over an unseen object, reflective clothing so you can be seen by others, and proper safety to reduce the chances of being mugged or assaulted.

Learning to play the game or sport properly is extremely important, which implies that the competitive rules will be followed. Rules serve various purposes, but one major purpose is to provide as safe and injury-free a situation as possible for that sport. Improper techniques are a major source of sports injuries. Poor body mechanics can place the individual in a most vulnerable position for injury. Landing on the wrong part of the foot when jogging and having the head in the wrong place when making a tackle in football are examples of improper body mechanics. The appropriate strategies for a sport must be learned. Having incorrect court or field position can place the individual in a precarious position for injury. As you gain experience, you learn to avoid certain situations that have high injury potential, and will develop a level of skill which will also provide a degree of protection. However, with experience comes repeated exposure, and with increased exposure comes an increased risk for injury. As an example, the longer one is on a football field in the heat of battle, the greater the opportunity for injury. The third-string quaterback who never gets into the game is at a very low risk for injury.

Having an *appropriate medical clearance* is, in reality, the first step in an injury prevention program. Screening out those individuals who are at a significant risk for injury is important. The prospective football player with bad knees, the recreational weight lifter with high blood pressure, and the long-distance runner who is diabetic should each receive special counsel, either encouraging them to seek another sport, or providing them with specific information that will allow them to compete at a lower risk. The medical examination should be designed for the sport. For the young football player, the examination should be heavily oriented toward the diagnosis of orthopedic problems or complications, while the examination for the middle-aged jogger should be oriented toward the diagnosis of respiratory and cardiovascular problems. For those 35 years of age and older, an exercise electrocardiogram is recommended.

Being properly conditioned for the sport is probably the most important factor in injury prevention. Many injuries are the result of simply not being prepared to handle the physical stress associated with the sport. Also, as a person begins to fatigue, the likelihood of injury increases, and there is a decrease in the ability to think as clearly, respond as quickly, move as rapidly, or hit as hard as was possible earlier in the activity. Being properly conditioned will not eliminate fatigue, but it will enable a person to handle considerably more physical stress before its onset, and will improve functioning under conditions of fatigue. Appropriate levels of strength and flexibility will prevent many musculoskeletal-types of injuries, and proper cardiorespiratory and muscular endurance will reduce those problems associated with fatigue. Finally, taking the time to stretch and warm up prior to exercise and competition will prevent many injuries.

Treatment of Injuries or Other Medical Problems

An injury should be treated just as soon as possible. Frequently, the length of time between the onset of injury and the initial stages of treatment can dictate the period of recovery and convalescence. For any injury of a potentially serious nature, such as head or eye injuries, fractures and chest pain, the individual and/or the specific part of the body that was injured should be immobilized. Standard first-aid procedures should be applied, and medical assistance should be obtained as quickly as possible. For injuries of a less serious nature, such as sprains, strains, and exposed wounds of a minor nature, immobilization, elevation, and ice is the usual sequence of treatments to follow. Compression of the injured area with an elastic bandage is also an effective treatment. Immobilization is necessary to prevent further damage and to reduce the pain associated with the injury. Elevation and ice are applied in an attempt to minimize and reduce swelling of or around the injured area. Once the situation has stabilized, the individual should seek medical attention. In the case of a suspected sprain, the physician may order an X ray to rule out the possibility of a fracture.

For overuse types of injuries, such as tendinitis, bursitis, shin splints, and bone bruises, frequently these will not require immediate medical attention. Rest and ice appear to be effective in the treatment of most overuse injuries; however, should the injury persist, medical consultation should be obtained. In most overuse types of injuries, the problem is compounded by the unwillingness of the individual to rest, and stay away from the stresses that caused the injury. Sometimes other activities of a less stressful nature, such as swimming and bicycling, can be substituted for the primary activity, allowing the individual to remain active while relieving the stresses associated with the primary activity. The jogger who develops a knee or ankle injury can possibly continue jogging by moving into the swimming pool in chest-deep water. The buoyancy force of the water considerably reduces the undesirable influence of gravity on the injury site, and allows exercise with minimal weight-bearing. Bicycling, either stationary or free cycling, also allow vigorous exercise without the stress of weight bearing.

Various treatment modalities are available to the individual at home which do not require special equipment or preparations. Over the past 10 years, one of the biggest breakthroughs in the treatment of athletic injuries has been the development of *cryokinetics*, or ice therapy. The immediate application of ice to an injury is now recognized as one of the most important aspects of the total treatment program. While the direct application of ice is initially painful, or at least uncomfortable, it does eventually reduce the direct pain resulting from the injury, relaxes the underlying muscles, reduces muscle spasms, and reduces surface blood flow while increasing deep blood flow, thus reducing swelling. Icing the injury will eventually lead to numbness of the surrounding area, and the injured joint can then be passively moved without pain throughout the complete range of motion. This passive-movement treatment should be used only when the possibility of a fracture or serious sprain has been ruled out.

Heat can also be used effectively in the long-term rehabilitation of an athletic injury, but not within the first 48 to 72 hours of injury. Heat increases local circulation and allows the underlying muscles to relax. Since heat can cause additional swelling, heat treatment should not be started until there has been a reduction in the initial swelling. When heat is used, wet heat appears to have a deeper, more penetrating effect. Hot, soaked towels, hydrocollator packs, hot baths, and whirlpools are good sources of wet heat.

Massage, taping, padding, and bracing are also helpful treatment modalities, but they should be used only by an individual who is trained in the use of these modalities, such as a physical therapist or an athletic trainer. Frequently, more harm than good can result when an individual undertakes a therapy program without appropriate advice and supervision.

At what point can the individual return to that activity in which the injury was sustained? For any serious injury, this is a decision which can be made only by the physician, therapist, or trainer who is familiar with the injury and has been involved in the rehabilitation program. It is much better to take a conservative approach at this point, for the premature return to the sport could result in a far more serious injury. For those injuries of a lesser nature, the individual should not return to the activity until the injured area is restored to its full range of motion, and until normal strength, power, and muscular endurance have been restored. The uninjured limb can be used as a comparison to the injured limb to determine the extent of full recovery. Movement should be free of hitches, limping, or any other abnormal or undesirable movement patterns. Finally, movement should be pain-free. Whenever pain is still present, the individual will have a tendency to favor that area, which can create additional problems in other parts of the body.

Most of the information presented in this section has been directed toward musculoskeletal injuries. There are also problems of a cardiovascular nature which must be considered. The participant must be aware of the various warning signs that may occur during or following strenuous exercise. Dr. Lenore Zohman, a prominent cardiologist in New York City, has devoted a number of years to the study of exercise prescription for the healthy as well as for those with specific cardiovascular diseases. In her booklet, "Beyond Diet . . .Exercise Your Way to Fitness and Heart Health," Dr. Zohman has listed a number of potential warning signs and symptoms that could occur during or immediately following exercise. These may be grouped into the following two categories:

A. Stop Exercising. See a physician before resuming.
1. Abnormal heart activity, including irregular pulse (missed beats or extra beats), fluttering, jumping, or palpitations

in the chest or throat, sudden burst of rapid heartbeats, or a sudden slowing of a rapid pulse rate

2. Pain or pressure in the center of the chest, or the arm or throat, during or immediately following exercise

3. Dizziness, lightheadedness, sudden lack of coordination, confusion, cold sweating, glassy stare, pallor, blueness, or fainting

4. Illness, particularly viral infections, can lead to myocarditis, inflammation of the heart muscle. Avoid exercise during and immediately following an illness.

B. Attempt Self-Correction.

1. Persistent rapid pulse rate throughout 5 to 10 minutes of recovery or longer
Self-Correction Technique: reduce the intensity of the activity (use a lower training heart rate) and progress to higher levels of activity at a slower rate. Consult a physician if the condition persists.

2. Nausea or vomiting after exercise
Self-Correction Technique: reduce the intensity of the endurance exercise and prolong the cool-down period. Avoid eating for at least 2 hours prior to the exercise session. Consult a physician if the condition persists.

3. Extreme breathlessness lasting more than 10 minutes after the cessation of exercise
Self-Correction Technique: reduce the intensity of the endurance exercise. Consult a physician if the condition persists.

4. Prolonged fatigue up to 24 hours following exercise
Self-Correction Technique: reduce the intensity of the endurance exercise and reduce the duration of the total workout session if this symptom persists. Consult a physician if these self-correcting techniques do not remedy the situation.

What is the potential for serious cardiovascular injury during exercise? James Fixx, runner and author of the best selling book, *The Complete Book of Running*, died of a heart attack while jogging during the summer of 1984. His death caused many to question the value of endurance exercise. First, how safe can it be if one of the leading proponents of exercise dies while jogging? Second, how can it possibly reduce the risk of death from coronary artery disease when he died of this disease in his mid-50s, a victim of his own beliefs? There is no question that anytime individuals participate in physical activity, they are going to be placing themselves in a higher risk situation than if they were to remain sedentary, but only for that particular point in time. With repeated bouts of exercise, as they become better conditioned they actually lower their risk for death from coronary artery disease, not only during that period of time during which they exercise, but throughout the entire 24-hour day. What about Jim Fixx? He was a very sedentary, overweight, cigarette smoking, overstressed executive in New York City until he reached his mid-30s. His father had died of a second heart attack in his early 40s, after suffering his first attack in his 30s. It was with the knowledge of his father's medical history and recognition of his own risk factors that Jim Fixx started running in his mid-30s. With his family history, and his own personal health history at that time, it is quite possible that he was able to prolong his life well beyond that which would have been expected had he elected to remain sedentary. Did Jim Fixx die prematurely as a result of his exercise program? Or did Jim Fixx add years to his life through his vigorous exercise program? Unfortunately, we will never know for certain, but the existing research in this field would certainly support the latter conclusion.

Bones and Muscles of the Body

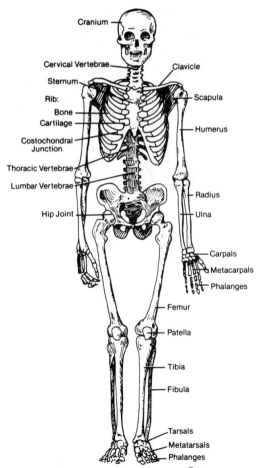

Figure 29 The human skeleton

Figure 30 Muscles of the body viewed from the front

Figure 31 Muscles of the body viewed from the rear

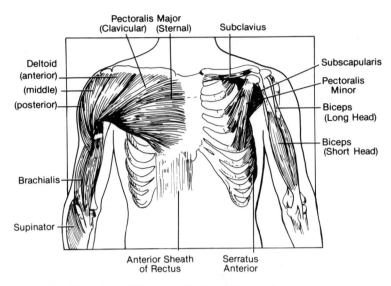

Figure 32   Muscles of the chest, shoulder, and arm

Figure 33   Muscles of the back, shoulder, and arm

Figure 34 Front view of the muscles of the arm and forearm

Figure 35 Rear view of the muscles of the forearm

Figure 36 Front view of the deep and superficial muscles of the lower extremity

Figure 37   Rear view of the deep and superficial muscles of the lower extremity

Metric Conversion Tables

Table 1 Equivalent Measures in Pounds (lbs) and Kilograms (kg)

lbs	kg	lbs	kg	lbs	kg
70	32	150	68	230	104
75	34	155	70	235	107
80	36	160	73	240	109
85	39	165	75	245	111
90	41	170	77	250	113
95	43	175	79	255	116
100	45	180	82	260	118
105	48	185	84	265	120
110	50	190	86	270	122
115	52	195	88	275	125
120	54	200	91	280	127
125	57	205	93	285	129
130	59	210	95	290	132
135	61	215	98	295	134
140	64	220	100	300	136
145	66	225	102		

Table 2   Equivalent Measures in Feet (ft) and Centimeters (cm)

ft, in	cm	ft	cm
3'	91	5'	152
3'2"	97	5'2"	157
3'4"	102	5'4"	163
3'6"	107	5'6"	168
3'8"	112	5'8"	173
3'10"	117	5'10"	178
4'	122	6'	183
4'2"	127	6'2"	188
4'4"	132	6'4"	193
4'6"	137	6'6"	198
4'8"	142	6'8"	203
4'10"	147	7'	213

Table 3   Equivalent Measures in Miles (mi) and Kilometers (km)

mi	km
3.1	5
6.2	10
9.3	15
12.4	20
15.5	25
18.6	30
21.7	35
24.8	40
28.0	45
31.0	50

Table 4 Equivalent Temperatures in Fahrenheit and Celsius

°F	°C
−40	−40
0	−18
32	0
50	10
72	22
85	30
98.6[1]	37
212	100

[1]Normal body temperature.

(The tables in this Appendix are adapted from Sharkey, B.J., 1984. *Physiology of fitness* (2nd ed.). Champaign, IL: Human Kinetics Publishers.)

References

American Heart Association. (1984). Report of Inter-Society Commission for Heart Disease Resources. *Circulation*, **70**, 157A-205A.

American Heart Association. (1986). *Heart facts*. Dallas, TX: Author.

Armstrong, R.B. (1984). Mechanisms of exercise-induced delayed onset muscular soreness: A brief review. *Medicine and Science in Sports and Exercise*, **16**, 529-538.

Bassler, T.J. (1975). Marathon running and immunity to heart disease. *Physician and Sportsmedicine*, **3**, 77-80.

Bray, G.A. (1979). Obesity in America. *International Journal of Obesity*, **3**, 363-375.

Cooper, K.H. (1968). A means of assessing maximal oxygen intake. *Journal of the American Medical Association*, **203**, 201-204.

Cooper, K.H., Pollock, M.L., Martin, R.P., White, S.R., Linnerud, A.C., & Jackson, A. (1976). Physical fitness levels vs. selected coronary risk factors: A cross-sectional study. *Journal of the American Medical Association*, **236**, 166-169.

DeLorme, T.L. (1945). Restoration of muscle power by heavy resistance exercises. *Journal of Bone and Joint Surgery*, **27**, 645-667.

DeLorme, T.L., & Watkins, A.L. (1948). Technics of progressive resistance exercise. *Archives of Physical Medicine*, **29**, 263-273.

deVries, H.A. (1980). *Physiology of exercise for physical education and athletics* (3rd ed.). Dubuque, IA: Wm. C. Brown.

Fahey, T. (1979). *What to do about athletic injuries*. New York: Butterick.

Food and Nutrition Board. (1980). *Recommended dietary allowances, ninth revised edition*. Washington, DC: National Research Council of the National Academy of Sciences.

Fox, E.L., & Mathews, D.K. (1974). *Interval training: Conditioning for sports and general fitness*. Philadelphia: W.B. Saunders.

Fox, S.M., III. (1969). Physical activity and coronary heart disease. *American Journal of Cardiology*, **23**, 298-303.

Getchell, L. (1979). *Physical fitness: A way of life* (2nd ed.). New York: John Wiley & Sons.

Gibbons, L.W., Blair, S.N., Cooper, K.H., and Smith, M. (1983). Association between coronary heart disease risk factors and physical fitness in healthy adult women. *Circulation*, **67**, 977-983.

Glasser, W. (1976). *Positive addiction*. New York: Harper and Row.

Hannon, B.M., & Lohman, T.G. (1978). The energy cost of overweight in the United States. *American Journal of Public Health*, **68**, 765-767.

Harris, Louis and Associates, Inc. (1979). *The Perrier Study: Fitness in America*. New York: Author.

Hettinger, T., & Müller, E.A. (1953). Muskellèistung und muskel training. *Arbèitsphysiologie*, **15**, 111-126.

Kannel, W.B., & Dawber, T.R. (1972). Atherosclerosis as a pediatric problem. *Journal of Pediatrics*, **80**, 544-554.

Kramsch, D.M., Aspen, A.J., Abramowitz, B.M., Kreimendahl, T., & Hood, W.B., Jr. (1981). Reduction of coronary atherosclerosis by moderate conditioning exercise in monkeys on an atherogenic diet. *New England Journal of Medicine*, **305**, 1483-1489.

Kraus, H., & Raab, W. (1961). *Hypokinetic disease*. Springfield, IL: Charles C. Thomas.

Metropolitan Life Insurance Company. (1959). New weight standards for men and women. *Statistical Bulletin Metropolitan Life Insurance Company*, **40**, 1-4.

Metropolitan Life Insurance Company. (1983). *1983 Metropolitan height and weight tables*. New York: Author.

Müller, E.A., & Rohmert, W. (1963). Die geschwindigkeit der muskelkraft-Zunahme bei isometrischem training. *Internationale Zeitschrift für Angewandte Physiologie einschliesslich Arbeitsphysiologie*, **19**, 403-419.

Multiple Risk Factor Intervention Trial Research Group (1982). Risk factor changes and mortality results. *Journal of the American Medical Association*, **248**, 1465-1477.

President's Council on Physical Fitness and Sports. (1972). *National Adult Physical Fitness Survey*. Princeton, NJ: Opinion Research Corporation.

President's Council on Physical Fitness and Sports. (January 1978). Sports potentials for physical fitness. *Physical Fitness Research Digest*, Series 8, #1.

Reisin, E., Abel, R., Modan, M., Silverberg, D.S., Eliahou, H.E., & Modan, B. (1978). Effect of weight loss without salt restriction on the reduction of blood pressure in overweight hypertensive patients. *New England Journal of Medicine*, **298**, 1-6.

Sharkey, B.J. (1984). *Physiology of fitness* (2nd ed.). Champaign, IL: Human Kinetics Publishers.

Wilmore, J.H. (1982). *Training for sport and activity* (2nd ed.). Boston: Allyn and Bacon.

Wilmore, J.H., & Bergfeld, J. (1979). A comparison of sports: Physiological and medical aspects. In R.H. Strauss (Ed.), *Sports medicine and physiology* (pp. 353-372). Philadelphia: W.B. Saunders.

Wind chill factor chart. (1973). *Runner's World*, **8**, 28.

Wood, P.D., & Haskell, W.L. (1979). The effect of exercise on plasma high density lipoproteins. *Lipids*, **14**, 417-427.

World Publications (Ed.). (1974). *The complete runner* (p. 306). Mountain View, CA: Author.

Zohman, L. (1974). *Beyond diet: Exercise your way to fitness and heart health*. Englewood Cliffs, NJ: Mazola Products, Best Foods. (Available through the local affiliate of the American Heart Association.)

Selected Readings

Part I

Optimal Health Through Physical Activity and Sport

Cardiovascular Disease

American College of Sports Medicine. (1985). *Guidelines for graded exercise testing and exercise prescription* (3rd ed.). Philadelphia: Lea & Febiger.

American Heart Association. (1980). *Heartbook: A guide to prevention and treatment of cardiovascular diseases.* Dallas: Author.

Amsterdam, E.A., Wilmore, J.H., & DeMaria, A.N. (Eds.). (1977). *Exercise in cardiovascular health and disease.* New York: Yorke Medical Books.

Cohen, L.S., Mock, M.B., & Ringqvist, I. (1981). *Physical conditioning and cardiovascular rehabilitation.* New York: John Wiley & Sons.

Ellestad, M.H. (1980). *Stress testing: Principles and practice* (2nd ed.). Philadelphia: F.A. Davis.

Farquhar, J.W. (1978). *The American way of life need not be hazardous to your health.* New York: W.W. Norton & Company.

Fletcher, G.F., & Cantwell, J.D. (1971). *Exercise in the management of coronary heart disease.* Springfield, IL: Charles C. Thomas.

Fletcher, G.F., & Cantwell, J.D. (1974). *Exercise and coronary heart disease.* Springfield, IL: Charles C. Thomas.

Franklin, B.A., & Rubenfire, M. (Eds.). (1984). *Clinics in sport medicine: Cardiac rehabilitation.* Philadelphia: W.B. Saunders.

Friedman, M., & Rosenman, R.H. (1974). *Type A behavior and your heart.* Greenwich, CT: Fawcett Crest Book, Fawcett Publications.

Froelicher, V.F. (1983). *Exercise testing and training.* New York: Le Jacq Publishing.

Gotto, A.M., Jr., et al. (1977). *Atherosclerosis.* Kalamazoo, MI: Upjohn.

James, W.E., & Amsterdam, E.A. (Eds.). (1977). *Coronary heart disease, exercise testing, and cardiac rehabilitation.* Miami, FL: Symposia Specialists Medical Books.

Kaplan, N.M., & Stamler, J. (Eds.). (1983). *Prevention of coronary heart disease: Practical management of the risk factors.* Philadelphia: W.B. Saunders.

Karvonen, M.J., & Barry, A.J. (Eds.). (1967). *Physical activity and the heart.* Springfield, IL: Charles C. Thomas.

Larsen, O.A., & Malmborg, R.O. (Eds.). (1971). *Coronary heart disease and physical fitness.* Baltimore: University Park Press.

Lauer, R.M., & Shekelle, R.B. (Eds.). (1980). *Childhood prevention of atherosclerosis and hypertension.* New York: Raven Press.

Little, R.C. (1977). *Physiology of the heart and circulation.* Chicago: Year Book Medical Publishers.

Long, C. (Ed.). (1980). *Prevention and rehabilitation in ischemic heart disease.* Baltimore: Williams & Wilkins.

Morse, R.L. (Ed.). (1972). *Excrcisc and the heart.* Springfield, IL: Charles C. Thomas.

Naughton, J.P., & Hellerstein, H.K. (Eds.). (1973). *Exercise testing and exercise training in coronary heart disease.* New York: Academic Press.

Opie, L.H. (1984). *Drugs for the heart.* New York: Grune and Stratton.

Polednak, A.P. (Ed.). (1979). *The longevity of athletes.* Springfield, IL: Charles C. Thomas.

Pollock, M.L., Wilmore, J.H., & Fox, S.M. (1984). *Exercise in health and disease: Evaluation and prescription for prevention and rehabilitation.* Philadelphia: W.B. Saunders.

Pollock, M.L., & Schmidt, D.H. (Eds.). (1979). *Heart disease and rehabilitation.* Boston: Houghton Mifflin.

Shephard, R.J. (1981). *Ischaemic heart disease and exercise.* Chicago: Year Book Medical Publishers.

Shepherd, J.T., & Vanhoutte, P.M. (1979). *The human cardiovascular system: Facts and concepts.* New York: Raven Press.

Sonnenblick, E.H., & Lesch, M. (Eds.). (1972). *Exercise and heart disease.* New York: Grune & Stratton.

Strong, W.B. (Ed.). (1978). *Atherosclerosis: Its pediatric aspects.* New York: Grune & Stratton.

Wenger, N.K. (Ed.). (1978). *Exercise and the heart.* Philadelphia: F.A. Davis.

Wenger, N.K., & Hellerstein, H.K. (Eds.). (1984). *Rehabilitation of the coronary patient* (2nd ed.). New York: John Wiley & Sons.

Wilson, P.K. (Ed.). (1975). *Adult fitness and cardiac rehabilitation*. Baltimore: University Park Press.

Wilson, P.K., Bell, C.W., & Norton, A.C. (1980). *Rehabilitation of the heart and lungs*. Fullerton, CA: Beckman Instruments.

Wilson, P.K., Fardy, P.S., & Froelicher, V.F. (1981). *Cardiac rehabilitation, adult fitness, and exercise testing*. Philadelphia: Lea & Febiger.

Obesity

Behnke, A.R., & Wilmore, J.H. (1974). *Evaluation and regulation of body build and composition*. Englewood Cliffs, NJ: Prentice-Hall.

Body Composition. (1963). *Annals of the New York Academy of Science*, **110**: Parts I and II.

Bray, G.A., & Bethune, J.E. (Eds.). (1974). *Treatment and management of obesity*. New York: Harper and Row.

Carter, J.E.L. (1980). *The Heath-Carter somatotype method* (3rd ed.). San Diego: San Diego State University.

Carter, J.E.L. (Ed.). (1982). *Physical structure of Olympic athletes*. New York: S. Karger.

Cioffi, L.A., James, W.P.T., & Van Itallie, T.B. (Eds.). (1981). *The body weight regulatory system: Normal and disturbed mechanisms*. New York: Raven Press.

Conn, H.L., Jr., DeFelice, E.A., & Kuo, P.T. (Eds.). (1983). *Health and obesity*. New York: Raven Press.

Craddock, D. (1978). *Obesity and its management* (3rd ed.). New York: Churchill Livingstone.

deGaray, A.L., Levine, L., & Carter, J.E.L. (1974). *Genetic and anthropological studies of Olympic athletes*. New York: Academic Press.

Garrow, J.S. (1978). *Energy balance and obesity in man* (2nd ed.). New York: Elsevier, North-Holland.

Greenwood, M.R.C. (Ed.). (1983). *Obesity*. New York: Churchill Livingstone.

Hansen, B.C. (Ed.). (1983). Controversies in obesity. *Endocrine and Metabolism Series*, **5**. New York: Praeger Publishers.

Katch, F.I., & McArdle, W.D. (1984). *Nutrition, weight control and exercise* (2nd ed.). Boston: Houghton Mifflin.

Mayer, J. (1972). *Human nutrition: Its physiological, medical, and social aspects*. Springfield, IL: Charles C. Thomas.

Munro, J.R. (Ed.). (1979). *The treatment of obesity*. Baltimore: University Park Press.

Nash, J.D., & Long, L.O. (1978). *Taking charge of your weight and well-being*. Palo Alto, CA: Bull Publishing.

National Institutes of Health. (1975). Obesity in perspective. *Fogarty International Center Series on Preventive Medicine*, (Vol. 2). Department of Health, Education, and Welfare #(NIH) 75-708.

Pařízková, J. (1977). *Body fat and physical fitness*. The Hague: Martinus Nijhoff B.V.

Powers, P.S. (1980). *Obesity: The regulation of weight*. Baltimore: Williams and Wilkins.

Storlie, J., & Jordon, H.A. (Eds.). (1984). *Nutrition and exercise in obesity management*. New York: Spectrum Publications.

Storlie, J., & Jordon, H.A. (Eds.). (1984). *Evaluation and treatment of obesity*. New York: Spectrum Publications.

Storlie, J., & Jordon, H.A. (Eds.). (1984). *Behavioral management of obesity*. New York: Spectrum Publications.

Stuart, R.B., & Davis, B. (1972). *Slim chance in a fat world*. Champaign, IL: Research Press.

Stunkard, A.J. (1980). *Obesity*. Philadelphia: W.B. Saunders.

Stunkard, A.J., & Stellar, E. (Eds.). (1984). *Eating and its disorders*. New York: Raven Press.

Tanner, J.M. (1964). *The physique of the Olympic athlete.* London: George Allen and Unwin.

Vague, J. (Ed). (1969). *Physiopathology of adipose tissue.* Amsterdam: Excerpta Medica Foundation.

Vague, J., & Boyer, J. (Eds.). (1974). *The regulation of the adipose tissue mass.* New York: American Elsevier Publishing.

Wilson, N.L. (Ed.). (1969). *Obesity.* Philadelphia: F.A. Davis.

Winick, M. (Ed.). (1975). *Childhood obesity.* New York: John Wiley & Sons.

Part II

The Prescription of Exercise for Fitness and Sport

Cooper, K.H. (1968). *Aerobics.* New York: M. Evans & Company.

Cooper, K.H. (1970). *The new aerobics.* New York: M. Evans & Company.

Cooper, K.H. (1977). *The aerobics way.* New York: M. Evans & Company.

Cooper, K.H. (1982). *The aerobics program for total well-being.* New York: M. Evans & Company.

Costill, D.L. (1979). A scientific approach to distance running. *Track and Field News.*

Daniels, J., Fitts, R., & Sheehan, G., (1978). *Conditioning for distance running.* New York: John Wiley & Sons.

Fahey, T.D. (1978). *The good-time fitness book.* New York: Butterick Publishing.

Faria, I.E., & Cavanagh, P.R. (1978). *The physiology and biomechanics of cycling.* New York: John Wiley & Sons.

Fixx, J.F. (1977). *The complete book of running*. New York: Random House.

Foss, M.L., & Garrick, J.G. (1978). *Ski conditioning*. New York: John Wiley & Sons.

Fox, E.L., & Mathews, D.K. (1974). *Interval training: Conditioning for sports and general fitness*. Philadelphia: W.B. Saunders.

Getchell, B. (1979). *Physical fitness: A way of life* (2nd ed.). New York: John Wiley & Sons.

Jensen, C.R., & Fisher, A.G. (1979). *Scientific basis of athletic conditioning* (2nd ed.). Philadelphia: Lea & Febiger.

Kuntzleman, C.T. (1975). *Activetics*. New York: Peter H. Wyden.

O'Shea, J.P. (1976). *Scientific principles and methods of strength fitness* (2nd ed.). Menlo Park, CA: Addison-Wesley.

Pollock, M.L., Wilmore, J.H., & Fox, S.M., III. (1978). *Health and fitness through physical activity*. New York: John Wiley & Sons.

Pollock, M.L., Wilmore, J.H., & Fox, S.M. (1984). *Exercise in health and disease: Evaluation and prescription for prevention and rehabilitation*. Philadelphia: W.B. Saunders Company.

Reid, J.G., & Thomson, J.M. (1985). *Exercise prescription for fitness*. Englewood Cliffs, NJ: Prentice-Hall.

Sharkey, B.J. (1984). *Physiology of fitness* (2nd ed.). Champaign, IL: Human Kinetics Publishers.

Stone, W.J., & Kroll, W.A. (1978). *Sports conditioning and weight training*. Boston: Allyn and Bacon.

Wilmore, J.H. (1982). *Training for sport and activity: The physiological basis of the conditioning process* (2nd ed.). Boston: Allyn and Bacon.

Part III

Special Considerations Related to Exercise and Sport

Albinson, J.G., & Andrew, G.M. (1976). *Child in sport and physical activity*. Baltimore: University Park Press.

American Association for Health, Physical Education and Recreation. (1971). *Nutrition for athletes*. Washington, DC: Author.

Bar-Or, O. (1983). *Pediatric sports medicine: From physiologic principles to clinical application*. New York: Springer Verlag.

Boileau, R.A. (Ed.). (1984). *Advances in pediatric sport sciences*, (Vol. 1). Champaign, IL: Human Kinetics Publishers.

Cooper, M., & Cooper, K.H. (1972). *Aerobics for women*. New York: M. Evans & Company.

Fahey, T.D. (1979). *What to do about athletic injuries*. New York: Butterick Publishing.

Katch, F.I., & McArdle, W.D. (1984). *Nutrition, weight control, and exercise* (2nd ed.). Boston: Houghton Mifflin.

Klafs, C.E., & Arnheim, D.D. (1969). *Modern principles of athletic training* (2nd ed.). St. Louis, MO: C.V. Mosby.

Klafs, C.E., & Lyon, M.J. (1973). *The female athlete*. St. Louis, MO: C.V. Mosby.

Miller, D.M. (1974). *Coaching the female athlete*. Philadelphia: Lea & Febiger.

Smith, N.J. (1976). *Food for sport*. Palo Alto, CA: Bull Publishing.

Smith, N.J., Ogilvie, B., Haskell, W., & Gaillard, B. (1978). *Handbook for the young athlete*. Palo Alto, CA: Bull Publishing.

Wells, C.L. (1985). *Women, sport and performance: A physiological perspective.* Champaign, IL: Human Kinetics Publishers.

Williams, M.H. (1976). *Nutritional aspects of human physical and athletic performance.* Springfield, IL: Charles C. Thomas.

Williams, M.H. (1983). *Nutrition for fitness and sport.* Dubuque, IA: Wm. C. Brown Publishers.

Young, D.R. (1977). *Physical performance, fitness and diet.* Springfield, IL: Charles C. Thomas.

Index

A

Abdomen, skinfold measurement, 23
Abrasions, 250
Adamson, G.T., 126
Air pollution, 211
Altitude, 209-211
Amenorrhea, 220
"American Exercise Survey," 120
American Heart Association, 11, 13
Amino acids, 233
Anemia, 63-65, 70
Angina pectoris, 8, 69, 245
Anxiety, 9, 33-34, 51-52
  causes of, 34
  combating, 51-52
  physical inactivity and, 33-34, 51-52
Aorta, 7
Ariel, Gidion, 149-150
Arthritis, types of, 34-35
Armstrong, R.B., 174
Aspartates, 247
Association of Physical Fitness Centers, 93
Atherosclerosis, 5-13
  stages of, 7-8

"Athlete's heart," 64
Athletic evaluation, 63-65
Athletic injuries, prevention and treatment, 249-263
  introduction to, 249
  medical problems associated with specific sports, 254-259
  prevention of injuries, 254-259
  treatment of injuries, 259-262
  types of injuries, 250-253

B

Back hyperextension, 105
Backward single leg raise, 106
Bar hang, 103
Basal metabolic rate (BMR), 222
Bassler, Thomas J., 43
Behind the neck press, 159
Bench-lying lateral arm raises, 170
Bench press, 160
Bent-arm pull-over, 164
Bent knee sit-up, 110
Bent rowing, 161

About The Author

Exercise is a common thread running through Jack Wilmore's life. He earned his PhD in physical education at the University of Oregon and is now a professor in the Department of Physical and Health Education at the University of Texas at Austin. Jack is the author of 12 books and more than 100 journal and magazine articles on various aspects of sports medicine and is a frequent consultant to many journals and organizations, including the President's Council on Physical Fitness and Sport.

Dr. Wilmore was recently appointed to the Sports Medicine Council of the U.S. Olympic Committee and chairs its research committee. He also frequently lectures throughout the country and conducts media tours for the National Dairy Council. An avid runner, Jack shares his enjoyment of an active life-style with his wife Dottie and their three daughters, Wendy, Kristi, and Melissa.